PATHOLOGY

MEDICAL EXAMINATION REVIEW

PATHOLOGY

Ninth Edition

600 Multiple-Choice Questions
with Referenced, Explanatory Answers

A. Olusegun Fayemi, M.D.

Associate Clinical Professor of Pathology
Mount Sinai School of Medicine of the City University of New York
New York

Director of Pathology and Laboratories
Interfaith Medical Center
Brooklyn, New York

MEDICAL EXAMINATION PUBLISHING COMPANY

No responsibility is assumed by the publisher for any injury and/or damage to persons or property as a matter of products liability, negligence or otherwise, or from any use or operation of any methods, products, instructions or ideas contained in the material herein. No suggested test or procedure should be carried out unless, in the reader's judgment, its risk is justified. Because the drugs specified within this book may not have specific approval by the Food and Drug Administration in regard to the indications and dosages that are recommended by the authors, we recommend that independent verification of diagnoses should be made. Discussions, views and recommendations as to medical procedures, choice of drugs and drug dosages are the responsibility of the authors.

Medical Examination Publishing Company
A Division of Elsevier Science Publishing Co., Inc.
52 Vanderbilt Avenue, New York, New York 10017

©1988 by Elsevier Science Publishing Co., Inc.

Library of Congress Cataloging-in-Publication Data

Medical examination review.
    Includes various editions of some volumes.
    Published 1960 – 1980 as: Medical examination review book.
    Includes bibliographical references.

    1. Medicine—Examinations, questions, etc.
RC58.M4   610'.76—dc19   61-66847   AACR 2   MARC

ISBN 0-444-01302-4

Current printing (last digit)
10 9 8 7 6 5 4 3 2 1

Manufactured in the United States of America

Contents

Preface

This ninth edition of *Pathology* has been substantially revised and updated to keep in step with current trends in medical education and the continuing expansion of scientific knowledge. It is designed to help prepare for course examinations, National Boards Part I, the Federation Licensing Examination (FLEX), and examinations for foreign medical graduates.

The range of subjects included in this volume is based on the content outline of the National Board of Medical Examiners, which develops the question pool for the tests mentioned above, and reflects the scope and depth of what is taught in medical schools today. The questions themselves are organized in broad categories to give you a representative sampling of the material covered in course work, while helping you define those general areas to which you need to devote attention. For your convenience in selective study, the answers (with commentary and references) follow each section of questions.

Each question has been scrutinized by specialists to verify that it is relevant and current. The author's care in item construction gives you questions that will provide good practice in familiarizing yourself with the format of objective-type tests. Questions of each type—one best response, matching, multiple true-false, and so on—are grouped together. They are modeled as closely as possible after those used by the Board.

Using this book, you may identify areas of strength and weakness in your own command of the subject. Specific references to widely used textbooks allow you to return to the authoritative source for further study. This volume supplements the lettered answers with brief explanations intended to prompt you to think about the choices — correct and incorrect—to put the answers in broadened perspective, and to add to your fund of knowledge. A complete bibliography appears at the end of the book. The questions and answers, taken together, emphasize problem solving and application of underlying principles as well as retention of factual knowledge.

1 General Pathology

DIRECTIONS: Each of the questions or incomplete statements below is followed by five suggested answers or completions. Select the one that is best in each case.

1. Cellular effects of hypoxic injury include all of the following EXCEPT
   A. loss of ATP
   B. depletion of glycogen
   C. increased activity of phosphofructokinase
   D. loss of intracellular sodium into the extracellular space
   E. cellular swelling

2. Prostaglandins E_1 and E_2 have been postulated as participating in which of the following regarding the process of inflammation?
   A. Chemotaxis
   B. Pavementing of leukocytes
   C. Vasodilatation
   D. Emigration of leukocytes
   E. None of the above

3. The symptom complex of dermatitis, dementia, and diarrhea is strongly suggestive of a deficiency of
    A. nicotinamide
    B. folic acid
    C. vitamin C
    D. riboflavin
    E. none of the above

4. Beriberi (thiamine deficiency) typically shows all of the following features EXCEPT
    A. confusion, ataxia, ophthalmoplegia (Wernicke's syndrome)
    B. posterolateral degeneration of the spinal cord
    C. congestive heart failure
    D. Korsakoff's psychosis
    E. fatty degeneration of myelin sheath

5. The digestive functions of the cell reside in the
    A. mitochondria
    B. lysosomes
    C. ribosomes
    D. Golgi complex
    E. endoplasmic reticulum

6. Which of the cellular organelles is involved with phagocytosis of bacteria and accumulation of cell debris?
    A. Phagosomes
    B. Lysosome
    C. Ribosome
    D. Endoplasmic reticulum
    E. Mitochondria

7. Immunologic deficiencies may be observed in association with all of the following EXCEPT
    A. multiple myeloma
    B. lymphomas
    C. lymphatic leukemia
    D. acute hepatic failure
    E. widespread cutaneous lesions

8. Atrophy is most strikingly characterized by
    A. fewer myofilaments
    B. fewer mitochondria
    C. less smooth endoplasmic reticulum
    D. less rough endoplasmic reticulum
    E. a greater number of autophagic vacuoles

9. Deposits of amyloid in whole organs can be diagnosed by staining the cut surfaces with
    A. Congo red
    B. PAS
    C. methylviolet
    D. iodine and dilute sulfuric acid
    E. toluidine blue

10. Histologically, amyloid deposits always begin
    A. intercellularly, often closely adjacent to the basement membrane
    B. intranuclearly, usually closely apposed to the nuclear membrane
    C. intracytoplasmically, enclosing the mitochondria
    D. intraglandularly, with close adherence to the epithelial lining
    E. intravascularly, with the venules and capillaries as the sites of predilection

11. Which of the following proteins is most likely to be found in a vasculitis of immune origin?
    A. Fibrin
    B. Alpha globulins
    C. Complement
    D. Gamma globulins
    E. Albumin

12. Which of the following has no bearing on the vascular changes observed in an anaphylactoid reaction?
    A. Serotonin
    B. Histamine
    C. Histones
    D. Kinins
    E. SRS (slow-reacting substance)

13. Which of the following cell types is most crucial in chronic rejection reaction?
    A. Lymphocytes
    B. Plasma cells
    C. Histiocytes
    D. Tissue eosinophils
    E. Segmented leukocytes

14. The most specific test for systemic lupus erythematosus is the demonstration of
    A. LE cells
    B. increased titers of ANA
    C. antibodies to double-stranded DNA
    D. increased titers of anti-RNA
    E. increased titers of antismooth muscle antibodies

15. Which of the following terms is least likely to metastasize?
    A. Glioblastoma multiforme
    B. Neuroblastoma
    C. Hepatoma
    D. Synovial sarcoma
    E. Leiomyoblastoma

16. Immunoglobulin specificity resides in the
    A. secondary folding of the molecule
    B. tertiary folding of the molecule
    C. genetic programming of the Fc fragment
    D. genetic programming of the Fab fragment
    E. precise amino acid sequence in the heavy chains

17. Rich iron deposits in the liver would be an unanticipated finding in which of the following?
    A. Alcoholic liver disease
    B. Idiopathic hemochromatosis
    C. After multiple blood transfusions
    D. Biliary cirrhosis
    E. Excessive dietary intake of iron

18. Serious hepatic functional deficit may NOT be observed in which of the following?
    A. Hepatic amyloidosis
    B. Alpha-l-antitrypsin deficiency
    C. Ingestion of extracts of senecio leaves
    D. Gaucher's disease
    E. von Gierke's disease

19. In which of the following rickettsial diseases is the human body louse the vector?
    A. Q fever
    B. Rickettsial pox
    C. Rocky Mountain spotted fever
    D. Epidemic typhus
    E. African tick typhus

20. Primary amebic meningoencephalitis is associated with
    A. eating raw fruits
    B. swimming in brackish or fresh water
    C. aerosolized droplet infection
    D. intestinal amebiasis
    E. insect bites

21. Which of the following is NOT characteristically seen in congenital toxoplasmosis?
    A. Diffuse encephalitis
    B. Granulomatous lesions of the leptomeninges
    C. Hydrocephalus
    D. Chorioretinitis
    E. Radiological opacities in the skull film

22. *Pneumocystis carinii* characteristically causes
    A. lobar pneumonia
    B. bronchopneumonia
    C. interstitial pneumonia with foamy intra-alveolar exudate
    D. pulmonary abscesses
    E. desquamative interstitial pneumonia

23. Primary amebic meningoencephalitis is usually caused by
  A. *Entamoeba coli*
  B. *Entamoeba histolytica*
  C. *Endolimax nana*
  D. *Acanthamoeba castellani*
  E. *Iodamoeba buetschlii*

24. "Sulfur granules" are characteristically present in infections by
  A. *Nocardia asteroides*
  B. *Actinomyces israelii*
  C. *Blastomyces dermatitidis*
  D. *Sporotrichum schenkii*
  E. *Histoplasma capsulatum*

25. The Frei test may be used in the diagnosis of
  A. toxoplasmosis
  B. *Pneumocystis carinii*
  C. lymphogranuloma venereum
  D. granuloma inguinale
  E. dengue fever

26. Which of the following is the most specific test in the diagnosis of syphilis?
  A. Complement fixation test
  B. Flocculation (VDRL)
  C. Darkfield microscopy
  D. Fluorescent antibody absorption test
  E. Rapid plasma reagent (RPR) test

27. Lymphogranuloma inguinale is synonymous with
  A. granuloma inguinale
  B. a disease caused by *Donovania granulomatis*
  C. lymphogranuloma venereum
  D. a disease in which LD bodies are found
  E. a disease caused by a bacterium

28. Lepra cells, found in lepromatous leprosy, are
    A. neutrophils
    B. lymphocytes
    C. histiocytes
    D. plasma cells
    E. fibroblasts

29. The Ghon's focus is located in which part of the lung?
    A. The apex
    B. The hilus
    C. The lower part of the upper lobes
    D. The diaphragmatic surface of the lung
    E. The pleural surface

30. A patient with a fever of 103°F, bradycardia, and leukopenia probably has
    A. brucellosis
    B. typhoid
    C. malaria
    D. melioidosis
    E. impetigo contagiosa

31. The primary site of proliferation of rickettsial organisms is in the
    A. parenchymal cells of the liver
    B. endothelial cells of small vessels
    C. media of arteries
    D. endothelial cells of large vessels
    E. adventitia of all blood vessels

32. Which of the following is NOT usually transmitted to man by arthropods?
    A. Scrub typhus
    B. Epidemic typhus
    C. Rocky Mountain spotted fever
    D. Endemic typhus
    E. Q fever

33. Negri bodies are located primarily in the
    A. astrocytes
    B. oligodendroglia
    C. neurons
    D. microglia
    E. ependymal cells

34. The most prominent pathological changes in poliomyelitis
    are in
    A. the posterior horn of the spinal cord
    B. the anterior horn of the spinal cord
    C. the spinal nerves
    D. the spinal ganglia
    E. none of the above

35. Which of the following is most resistant to gonococcal infec-
    tion?
    A. Anterior urethra
    B. Posterior urethra
    C. Epididymis
    D. Prostate
    E. Testis

36. Which of the following is considered the predominant micro-
    bicidal system in phagocytic cells?
    A. Lactoferrin
    B. Lysozyme
    C. Phagocytin
    D. H_2O_2-halide ion
    E. Elastase

37. Primary causes of noninflammatory edema include all of the
    following EXCEPT
    A. an increase in intravascular hydrostatic pressure
    B. increased vascular permeability
    C. diminished plasma colloid osmotic pressure
    D. lymphatic obstruction
    E. an impairment of renal function

38. Probable pathogenetic mechanisms that have been postulated to operate in septic shock include all of the following EXCEPT
   A. increased peripheral vascular resistance
   B. venoconstriction
   C. direct toxic endothelial injury
   D. activation of complement
   E. release of interleukin 1 from macrophages

39. The vast majority of patients with primary gout reveal
   A. normal production of uric acid with reduced excretion
   B. a lack of hypoxanthine-guanine phosphoribosyl transferase
   C. overproduction of uric acid with increased excretion
   D. overproduction of uric acid with normal excretion
   E. overproduction of uric acid with tissue storage of uric acid

40. A lack or deficiency of a lysosomal enzyme is the basis for all the following EXCEPT
   A. type 2 glycogenosis (Pompe's disease)
   B. Tay Sach's disease
   C. Gaucher's disease
   D. type 1 glycogenosis (von Gierke's disease)
   E. Mucopolysaccharidosis type 1 (Hurler's syndrome)

41. The most prevalent pulmonary infection in patients with acquired immunodeficiency syndrome (AIDS) is caused by
   A. *Candida albicans*
   B. *Cryptococcus neoformans*
   C. *Toxoplasma gondi*
   D. *Pneumocystis carinii*
   E. *Cytomegalovirus*

42. A localized overgrowth of mature cells in a tissue resembling, or having some features, of a tumor most closely describes
    A. desmoplasia
    B. metaplasia
    C. choriostoma
    D. hamartoma
    E. anaplasia

43. Dysplasia is characterized by all of the following EXCEPT
    A. disorderly proliferation of cells
    B. pleomorphism
    C. hyperchromaticity
    D. most frequently occurs in epithelium
    E. relentless progression to malignant neoplasm

DIRECTIONS: For each of the questions or incomplete statements below, **one** or **more** of the answers or completions given is correct. Select

    A if only *1, 2, and 3* are correct
    B if only *1 and 3* are correct
    C if only *2 and 4* are correct
    D if only *4* is correct
    E if all are correct

---

44. The component(s) of complement system that has (have) biologic activity in inflammation is (are)
    1. C4
    2. C3a
    3. C2
    4. C567

45. Rickets in children and/or osteomalacia in adults have been described in
    1. Fanconi syndrome
    2. renal tubular acidosis
    3. chronic malabsorption disorders
    4. nutritional deficiency of vitamin D

46. Autoimmune pathogenic mechanisms seem to play a role in
    1. experimental foreign protein nephritis
    2. human serum sickness nephritis
    3. postpneumococcal glomerulonephritis
    4. lupus nephritis

47. The antibody(ies) found in the sera of patients with systemic lupus erythematosus include(s)
    1. anti-RNA
    2. anti-DNA
    3. anti-Sm
    4. anti-nucleoprotein

48. Visual difficulties encountered following exposure to methyl alcohol may be related to
    1. a defect in synthesis of ATP
    2. interference with glucose metabolism
    3. arrest of retinal hexokinase activity
    4. advanced fatty change in neurons of retina

49. The deleterious effect(s) of exposure to carbon monoxide include(s)
    1. cumulative effect
    2. a strong affinity for hemoglobin
    3. system asphyxiation
    4. a strong irritant effect

50. Hemochromatosis is characterized by
    1. pigment cirrhosis
    2. siderosis of other organs
    3. pancreatic fibrosis and siderosis
    4. pigmentation of the skin

51. The smooth, or agranular, endoplasmic reticulum (SER) is involved in the
    1. synthesis of lipids
    2. conjugation of bile pigments
    3. conduction of contractile impulses
    4. detoxification of many drugs and chemical agents

Directions Summarized				
A	B	C	D	E
1,2,3	1,3	2,4	4	All are
only	only	only	only	correct

52. When the components of the complement system interact they
    1. promote phagocytosis of particles and organisms by opsonization and coating of these aggregates
    2. yield chemotactic factors that direct the migration of polymorphonuclear leukocytes
    3. yield anaphylatoxins
    4. cause cell membrane damage in red blood cells

53. The characteristic gross pattern(s) of splenic amyloidosis is (are)
    1. marked collagenous thickening or "sugar coating" of splenic capsule
    2. enlarged; tapioca-like granules largely limited to the splenic follicles
    3. markedly enlarged; firm, dark-red meaty parenchmya with small gray-to-brown nodules scattered throughout the red pulp
    4. enlarged; pale, map-like areas of increased consistency at first limited to the pulp

54. In amyloidosis, the kidney, on gross inspection, may appear
    1. normal in size and color
    2. enlarged; pale gray and firm
    3. shrunken and contracted
    4. faintly nodular owing to cortical subcapsular masses of amyloid

55. Cancer(s) with a propensity for venous invasion is (are)
    1. adenocarcinoma of breast
    2. renal cell carcinoma
    3. leiomyosarcoma
    4. hepatocarcinoma

56. The factor(s) involved in the loss of cohesion in cancerous tissues is (are)
1. less calcium content of cancerous tissues as compared to normal tissues
2. failure of epithelial surface cancers to form intercellular junctions
3. increased repulsive electrical charges between cells
4. invariable presence of phagocytic cells with subsequent piecemeal fragmentation of the neoplastic mass

57. Which of the following tumors appear(s) to have hormone-dependent growth increase?
1. Fibroadenoma of breast
2. Uterine leiomyoma
3. Prostatic adenocarcinoma
4. Choriocarcinoma of testes

58. The capsule of a benign neoplasm is produced by
1. fibrous tissue elaborated by native parenchyma
2. atrophy of the surrounding normal parenchymal cells, caused by the pressure of a growing mass
3. ischemic necrosis followed by scar formation at the periphery of the new growth when it outspaces its blood supply
4. stroma of the tumor itself

59. Which of the following is (are) most capable of hypertrophy?
1. Striated muscle cells of the heart
2. Smooth muscle cells of the media of medium-sized arteries
3. Striated muscle cells of the skeletal muscles
4. Smooth muscle cells of the gastrointestinal wall

60. Intracellular accumulations of lipid are seen in
1. atherosclerosis
2. lesions of traumatic fat necrosis
3. certain forms of glomerular disease
4. xanthomas

		Directions Summarized		
A	B	C	D	E
1,2,3	1,3	2,4	4	All are
only	only	only	only	correct

61. Intracellular accumulations of protein are seen in
    1. plasma cells
    2. diabetes mellitus
    3. nephrotic syndrome
    4. Pompe's disease

62. The endogenous pigment(s) NOT derived from hemoglobin is (are)
    1. hemosiderin
    2. lipofuscin
    3. hematin
    4. melanin

63. Reduced capacity for rejection of graft is encountered principally in
    1. Hashimoto's thyroiditis
    2. sarcoidosis
    3. tuberculosis
    4. Hodgkin's disease

64. Which of the following is (are) prototype immune response(s) to exogenous antigen?
    1. Arthus phenomenon
    2. Serum sickness
    3. Anaphylaxis
    4. Tuberculin reaction

65. Hypertrophy and hyperplasia are found in
    1. the left kidney after a right nephrectomy
    2. the left ventricle of a patient with aortic stenosis
    3. gravid uterus
    4. skeletal muscles of a laborer engaged in heavy work

66. Meningococcal colonization of the mucous membrane of the upper respiratory tract may result in?
    1. carrier state
    2. meningococcemia
    3. meningitis
    4. formation of hemagglutinating antibodies

67. Which of the following bacteremic states is (are) associated with skin manifestations?
    1. Meningococcemia
    2. Secondary syphilis
    3. Rickettsial diseases
    4. Typhoid fever

68. Heterophile-negative infectious mononucleosis may be associated with
    1. cytomegalovirus
    2. toxoplasmosis
    3. infectious hepatitis
    4. ingestion of certain drugs

69. Which of the following produce(s) granulomas which may be difficult to distinguish from a tubercle?
    1. Berylliosis
    2. Histoplasmosis
    3. Syphilis
    4. Boeck's sarcoid

70. *Listeria monocytogenes* is associated with
    1. myocardial necrosis
    2. repeated spontaneous abortion and stillbirths
    3. multiple organ abscesses
    4. meningoencephalitis

71. Rat-bite fever may be caused by
    1. *Leptospira canicola*
    2. *Streptobacillus moniliformis*
    3. *Borrellia recurrentis*
    4. *Spirillum minus*

Directions Summarized

A	B	C	D	E
1,2,3	1,3	2,4	4	All are
only	only	only	only	correct

72. Typical clinical manifestation(s) of Q fever include(s)
    1. pneumonia
    2. diffuse maculopapular rash
    3. granulomatous hepatitis
    4. meningoencephalitis

73. Lymphogranuloma inguinale
    1. is a malignant disease of the lymph nodes
    2. morphologically resembles cat-scratch disease
    3. is caused by an oncogenic virus
    4. may cause elephantiasis of the external genitalia

74. Cat-scratch disease
    1. is always caused by cats
    2. is most common in childhood
    3. morphologically shows sarcoid-like granulomas
    4. is predominantly a disease of the lymph nodes

75. *Entamoeba histolytica* infection may involve the
    1. colon
    2. skin
    3. liver
    4. brain

76. In which of the following would opportunistic fungal infections occur?
    1. Diabetes mellitus
    2. Leukemia
    3. Patients on immunosuppressive therapy
    4. Malignant lymphoma

77. Concerning plague, it may be said that the
   1. most common form is the pneumonic form
   2. organisms excite a granulomatous reaction in the lung
   3. disease is never transmitted from person to person
   4. disease is generally transmitted by the bite of *Xenopsylla cheopis*

78. Zenker's hyaline necrosis of skeletal muscle may occur secondary to
   1. physical trauma
   2. sudden ischemia
   3. extremes of temperature
   4. typhoid fever

79. Which of the following statement(s) is (are) true regarding legionella infection?
   1. The causative organisms are gram negative, flagellated, and are best visualized by immunofluorescence
   2. The disease may manifest as Pontiac fever, a self-limited febrile illness
   3. Pulmonary involvement takes the form of confluent bronchopneumonia, which histologically reveals a high mononuclear-to-neutrophil ratio
   4. Infections caused by the organism are prevalent in premature infants and chronic hemodialysis patients

80. The infectious agent of cytomegalic inclusion disease has been shown to be spread through
   1. intrauterine transmission to the fetus
   2. transplantation of organs of patients with latent infection
   3. venereal transmission
   4. blood transfusions

81. Which of the following is (are) considered physiologic hyperplasia?
   1. Cystic endometrial hyperplasia
   2. Hyperplasia of the glandular epithelium of the breast of pubertal and pregnant females
   3. Adenomatous endometrial hyperplasia
   4. Proliferative endometrium

Directions Summarized				
A	B	C	D	E
1,2,3	1,3	2,4	4	All are
only	only	only	only	correct

82. Which of the following changes may be seen in cellular adaptation?
    1. Hypertrophy
    2. Hyperplasia
    3. Metaplasia
    4. Dysplasia

83. Hypoxic injury may occur in
    1. carbon monoxide poisoning
    2. cyanide poisoning
    3. embolic arterial occlusion
    4. severe arteriosclerosis

84. Increased permeability of venules during the acute inflammatory process is mediated by which of the following?
    1. Bradykinin
    2. Leukotriene C_4
    3. Histamine
    4. Prostaglandin E_2 (PGE2)

85. Marfan's syndrome, an autosomal disorder of defective collagenous and elastic fiber formation, is characterized by
    1. a primary defect in the organization of elastic fibers
    2. mutation of the pro-alpha 2 (I) gene
    3. genetic heterogeneity
    4. inhibition of the cross-linking enzyme lysyl oxidase

86. Down's syndrome may be associated with which of the following chromosomal abnormalities?
    1. Translocation
    2. Trisomy
    3. Mosaicism
    4. Deletion

87. Which of the following immunological derangements is (are) associated with acquired immunodeficiency syndrome (AIDS)?
    1. Inversion of T4(helper)/T8 (suppressor) ratio
    2. Selective destruction of OKT4 lymphocytes
    3. Impairment of blast transformation in in vitro tests
    4. Elevated levels of serum immunoglobulins

88. Human immunodeficiency virus (HIV)
    1. is a nontransforming cytopathic retrovirus
    2. possesses genomic RNA
    3. shows selective tropism for T4 helper/inducer lymphocytes
    4. has been shown to also infect B lymphocytes

89. Squamous metaplastic changes may occur in the epithelium of which of the following?
    1. Bronchus
    2. Urinary bladder
    3. Endocervix
    4. Gall bladder

90. A high propensity for venous invasion is found in which of the following neoplasms?
    1. Renal cell carcinoma
    2. Breast carcinoma
    3. Hepatocellular carcinoma
    4. Colonic carcinoma

DIRECTIONS: Each group of questions below consists of lettered headings followed by a list of numbered words, phrases, or statements. For **each** numbered word, phrase, or statement, select the **one** lettered heading that is most closely associated with it. Each lettered heading may be selected once, more than once, or not at all.

Questions 91–95:
    A. Immunoblasts
    B. B lymphocytes
    C. T lymphocytes

91. Transformed lymphocytes committed to respond to only one antigen

92. Subcortical and paracortical in lymph nodes; periarteriole sheaths in spleen

93. Cortical, about the follicles in lymph nodes and spleen; diffuse throughout marrow

94. Constitute most of the lymphocytes in the circulating blood

95. Large pyroninophilic cells with abundant ribosomes and polyribosomes

Questions 96–102:
    A. Tuberculin reaction
    B. Serum sickness
    C. Anaphylaxis
    D. Arthus reaction

96. Adsorption of IgE to specific membrane receptors on mast cells triggering the release of vasoactive compounds

97. Complement-mediated acute necrotizing angiitis with consequent damage to cells and tissues in the local area

98. Systemic immune disease caused by formation of small soluble antigen-antibody aggregates within the circulation

99. Prototype of cell-mediated response

100. Induced by intravenous injection of antibody followed by subcutaneous antigenic challenge

101. Rapidly developing immunologic reaction resulting from the combination of antigen and IgE

102. Mediation by T lymphocytes

Questions 103–109:
  A. NADPH
  B. Leukotriene B₄
  C. Prostaglandin (PGI₂)
  D. C3b
  E. Interleukin-1

103. Functions as an opsonin in the inflammatory process

104. A polypeptide and an endogenous pyrogen produced by macrophages

105. Chediak-Higashi syndrome

106. Potent vasodilator

107. Chemotaxis and aggregation of neutrophils

108. Involved in microbicidal activity in phagocytes

109. Potentiates margination

Questions 110–117:
  A. *Trichophyton rubrum*
  B. *Cryptococcus neoformans*
  C. *Coccidioides immitis*
  D. *Sporothrix schenckii*
  E. *Rhizopus* sp.

110. Diabetic acidosis; ophthalmoplegia; diffuse cerebrovascular disease

111. Slow-to-heal ulcer on hand; string of secondary chancroid ulcers; regional lymphadenopathy

112. Alcoholic gardeners are highly susceptible to infection

113. Lesions may be mistaken for mucin-secreting carcinoma

114. Cavitary or solid "coin" lesions of lung

115. Mucicarmine stain

116. Thick-walled spherule containing numerous endospores

117. Onychomycosis

Questions 118–123:
- A. *Bordetella pertussis*
- B. *Corynebacterium diphtheriae*
- C. *Neisseria gonorrhoeae*
- D. *Candida albicans*
- E. *Cryptococcus neoformans*

118. Thayer-Martin agar

119. Chlamydospore

120. Bordet-Gengou medium

121. Tellurite blood agar

122. India ink preparation

123. Sabourad's dextrose broth

Questions 124 – 128:
- A. *Aspergillus fumigatus*
- B. *Cryptococcus neoformans*
- C. *Coccidiodes immitis*
- D. *Cryptosporidium*
- E. *Entamoeba histolytica*
- F. *Histoplasma capsulatum*
- G. *Mucormycosis*

124. Intracellular 2- to 5-µm, round to ovoid bodies, demonstrable by hematoxylin and eosin and silver stain

125. Gelatinous capsule demonstrable by India ink

126. Bronchial asthma of type III and type IV hypersensitivity reaction

127. Encountered most commonly in patients with diabetic ketoacidosis, immunodeficiency, and advanced malignancy. Nonseptate, broad hyphae with marked right angle branching

128. Chronic and debilitating diarrhea in patients with immunodeficiency. Microgametes and macrogametes arranged along brush border of gut epithelium

---

DIRECTIONS: The set of lettered headings below is followed by a list of numbered words or phrases. For each numbered word or phrase select

A   if the item is associated with (A) *only*
B   if the item is associated with (B) *only*
C   if the item is associated with *both* (A) *and* (B)
D   if the item is associated with *neither* (A) *nor* (B)

Questions 129–134:
A. Marasmus
B. Kwashiorkor
C. Both
D. Neither

129. State of malnutrition in which there is a deficiency of total calories

130. Fatty liver

131. Associated with depressed T- and B-cell functions

132. Characteristic skin lesions

133. Normochromic normocytic anemia

134. Peripheral neuropathy

Questions 135–141:
   A. RNA oncogenic virus
   B. DNA oncogenic virus
   C. Both
   D. Neither

135. Reverse transcriptase

136. Human papilloma virus

137. Cancer induction involves association of viral genome with genome of host cells

138. V-oncogene

139. HTLV-1

140. Transformed host cell cannot replicate more virus

141. Proto-oncogene

Answers and Comments

1. D. Decrease of oxygen tension within the cell (hypoxia) leads to loss of oxidative phosphorylation associated with loss of ATP production which in turn, causes sodium to accumulate intracellularly and potassium to diffuse out of the cell. The net cellular solute gain is accompanied by isoosmotic gain of water and consequent cell swelling. (REF. 1, pp. 5–9)

2. C. PGE_1 and PGE_2 are potent vasodilators and contribute to edema formation during the process of inflammation by potentiating the vascular permeability effects of other mediators. Prostaglandin production may also be one of the causes of fever during inflammatory reactions. (REF. 1, p. 56)

3. A. The symptom complex describes pellagra, the result of a deficiency of nicotinamide. The dementia is caused by degeneration of ganglion cells of the brain as well as degeneration of tracts of the spinal cord. The dermatitis is usually symmetrical and often located in areas exposed to sunlight or chronic irritation. (REF. 1, pp. 415–416)

4. B. The heart in beriberi is characteristically flabby and dilated, more predominantly in the right than in the left side. Interstitial myocardial edema is the most consistent histopathologic change. A variety of nonspecific alterations of the peripheral and central nervous system have been described. The predominance of either the cardiac or nervous system disturbance or a combination of such signs forms the basis to the distinction between the "dry" or "wet" type of beriberi. (REF. 1, p. 413)

5. B. Lysosomes are reservoirs of digestive enzymes that are separated in membrane-bound sacs in healthy cells. During cellular injury, lysosomes are disrupted, and the enzymes contained within are free for digestion of cellular substance. (REF. 1, p. 26)

6. A. Ribosomes and endoplasmic reticulum are involved with protein synthesis. Mitochondria are the seat of oxidative and reductive enzyme systems. Lysosomes are reservoirs of lytic enzymes. (REF. 1, pp. 13, 26)

7. D. Immunologic deficits are sometimes observed in association with lymphoproliferative disorders and plasma cell dyscrasias. The liver has no direct role in the integrity of immunologic mechanisms. (REF. 1, p. 691)

8. E. Autophagic vacuoles appear to form when breakdown of intracellular components and organelles occurs. Separation of damaged cell substance in the form of autophagic vacuoles appears as an adaptive response in atrophy. (REF. 1, p. 30)

9. D. Amyloid deposits in whole organs develop a mahogany brown color with iodine and dilute sulfuric acid. (REF. 1, p. 201)

10. A. Congo red staining followed by polarizing microscopy will often disclose trace amounts of amyloid not readily seen by light microscopy. With progression of the process, nodular masses of amyloid fuse, encroach on neighboring cells and, in time, entrap and destroy the cellular constituents of the involved organ. (REF. 1, p. 201)

11. D. The deposition of gamma globulins points to an immunologic pathogenic mechanism. (REF. 1, p. 169)

12. C. Histones are basic proteins that form an integral part of the DNA molecule. They have no vasoactive properties. (REF. 1, p. 281)

13. A. The phenomenon of delayed rejection reaction is mediated by immunologic mechanisms, and the lymphocyte is the critical cell type involved in chronic rejection reaction. Plasma cells and histiocytes are also frequently observed. (REF. 1, pp. 174–175)

14. C. To this date, antibodies to double-stranded DNA have only been reported in SLE. Increased ANA and positive LE cell test are found in 60-80% of patients with Sjögren's syndrome, 80% with scleroderma, and 15-25% with adult rheumatoid arthritis. (REF. 1, p. 181)

15. A. In the brain, the malignancy of a tumor must be thought of in two senses: the strategic importance of its location and the aggressiveness of its cellular constituents. (REF. 1, pp. 225–229)

16. D. The former view of the occurrence of secondary or tertiary folding of the immunoglobulin has been largely invalidated by the sequential amino acid analysis that has shown that specificity is conferred by the precise amino acids sequence and genetic programming of the variable portion of the polypeptide subunits of the immunoglobulin molecule. (REF. 3, p. 865)

17. D. Among the mechanisms invoked in the iron overload that complicates liver cirrhosis are excessive iron absorption, intrahepatic arteriovenous shunts, and derangements of iron metabolism. (REF. 1, pp. 925–926)

18. A. Alpha-1-antitrypsin deficiency has been associated with liver cirrhosis; hepatic veno-occlusive disease has been observed following ingestion of senecio alkaloids. In both Gaucher's and von Gierke's disease, there are accumulations of glucocerebrosides and glycogen respectively in the liver, with significant hepatomegaly and liver dysfunction. (REF. 1, pp. 204–205)

19. D. All the rickettsial diseases included in the choices with the exception of epidemic typhus are transmitted to man by ticks. Epidemic typhus occurs over most of the world in winter and spring, especially in cold climates. (REF. 1, p. 298)

20. B. This disease is caused by free living amebae, *Naegleria fowleri*, or less commonly by free living *Hartmanella* species of ameba. The route of entry is the nasopharyngeal mucosa. (REF. 1, p. 363)

21. A. Characteristically, the lesions involving the central nervous system in toxoplasmosis include destructive granulomatous lesions involving the leptomeninges, ependyma, superficial brain substance, and the eye. Also, calcification of these lesions is responsible for the typical opacities seen in the skull radiographs. (REF. 1, pp. 373–374)

22. C. The alveoli contain foamy eosinophilic exudate in which many organisms are demonstrable by special stains. (REF. 1, pp. 365–366)

23. D. The organism is also call *Hartmanella castellani*. Culture methods are available for body fluids and tissues. (REF. 1, p. 363)

24. B. The *Actinomyces* are weakly acid-fast and tend to grow in a colony formation within tissue lesions. They thus create a dense central mat of tangled threads called "sulfur granules." (REF. 1, pp. 349–350)

25. C. A positive Frei skin test is of limited significance, since it merely demonstrates the presence, or previous existence, of an infection. (REF. 1, pp. 294–295)

26. D. A new addition to the laboratory diagnosis of syphilis is the *Treponema pallidum* hemagglutination test. (REF. 3, pp. 1140–1142)

27. C. It is also called lymphopathia venereum and is transmitted by sexual intercourse. It is manifested in the acute stages by necrotizing lymphadenitis. (REF. 1, p. 862)

28. C. Lepra cells are lipid-laden and contain myriad organisms (globi). (REF. 1, pp. 347–348)

29. C. This is the primary lesion of primary tuberculosis. It may also be located at the upper part of the lower lobes in the subpleural areas. (REF. 1, pp. 343–344)

30. B. Typhoid characteristically shows a dissociation between the temperature and pulse rate—a high temperature is associated with a low pulse rate. The lack of neutrophilic infiltrate in typhoid lesions correlates with the leukopenia that is found. (REF. 1, pp. 319–321)

31. B. These organisms may be visualized in infected cells by Giemsa or Macchiavello stains. Their presence in endothelial cells is often followed by thrombosis of the vessels. (REF. 1, p. 295)

32. E. There is a strong suspicion that it may be transmitted to man without an animal or arthropod vector via infectious placentas of infected sheep or by inhalation. (REF. 2, p. 341)

33. C. Grossly the brain, spinal cord, and viscera show congestion and petechial hemorrhages. Other morphologic changes include demyelinization, focal ganglion cell degeneration, and perivascular lymphocytic infiltrate. (REF. 1, p. 1384)

34. B. The ganglion cells show chromatolysis and other degenerative changes. Inclusion bodies may be found in the early stages of the disease. (REF. 1, pp. 1384–1385)

35. E. Although gonococcal epididymitis is characteristic of neglected cases of gonorrhea, the testis is remarkably resistant. (REF. 1, pp. 309–310)

36. D. Lactoferrin, lysozyme, phagocytin, and elastase belong to the so-called oxygen-independent system and, although they participate in the killing of bacteria ingested by neutrophils and macrophages, the major microbicidal system is that which involves superoxide $O_2.-$, H_2O_2-halide ions, and the enzyme myeloperoxidase. (REF. 6, p. 36)

37. B. Increased vascular permeability contributes significantly to inflammatory edema and exudation in addition to increased hydrostatic pressure. The former is mediated in its early phases by histamine, serotonin, and bradykinin; contraction of endothelial cells with formation intercellular gaps, or a direct damage to the endothelial cells, also occurs during the inflammatory process. (REF. 6, p. 63)

38. A. Theories abound regarding the pathogenesis of septic shock. Most commonly observed in gram-negative and staphylococcal septicemia, it has also been described in pneumococcal septicemias. There is an inappropriate diminution of peripheral resistance due to arteriolar dilatation caused by direct toxic injury, release of complement components, kinins, and platelet products. (REF. 6, pp. 79–80)

39. C. The enzymatic defects that underlie the overproduction of uric acid in primary gout are unknown. In about 15% of patients, there is an enzymatic defect, principally of hypoxanthine-guanine phosphoribosyl and amidophosphoribosyl transferases. (REF. 6, p. 99)

40. D. Most of the lysosomal storage disorders are inherited as autosomal recessive traits. The enzyme deficiency in the various diseases are the following: Pompe's disease, lysosomal glucosidase; Tay Sach's disease, hexosaminidase A; Gaucher's disease, glucocerebroside; and Hurler's syndrome, alpha-L-iduronidase. (REF. 6, pp. 112–113)

41. D. Lung infection by *Pneumocystis carinii* occurs in about 50% of AIDS patients. Other opportunistic infections that commonly occur in these patients include herpes simplex, atypical mycobacteriosis, especially *Mycobacterium avium-intracellulare* and aspergillosis. (REF. 6, pp. 176–177)

42. D. Although the cells in a hamartoma are mature, benign, and nonneoplastic, there is abnormal organization of the cells so that the lesion does not resemble the normal tissue from which it is derived. The hamartoma is a type of congenital anomaly and not a neoplasm. (REF. 6, p. 188)

43. E. Most commonly observed in the uterine cervix, respiratory, and gastrointestinal tracts, dysplasia may be related to chronic inflammation or persistent irritation; an etiology is, however, not always identifiable. The lesion is potentially reversible if the source of irritation is eliminated. (REF. 6, p. 185)

44. C. C3a and C5a increase vascular permeability. C5a and C567 are chemotactic agents. (REF. 1, pp. 52–53)

45. E. Rickets and/or osteomalacia may also be caused by cholestatic liver disease, long-term anticoagulant therapy, and sex-linked hypophosphatemia. The basic alteration in this disorder is failure of mineralization of osteoid matrix with consequent excess of osteoid tissue in the bones. (REF. 1, pp. 406–408)

46. D. Lupus nephritis is considered an autoimmune disease. Exogenous antigens have not been involved in the pathogenesis of this disorder. Low levels of serum complement activity and deposits as seen in immunofluorescence studies of renal sections point to the presence of immune pathogenic mechanisms. (REF. 1, pp. 176–189)

47. E. A very large number of antibodies against self-constituents have been observed in systemic lupus erythematosus. All the four types of antibodies included here have been documented to be present in several instances of SLE. (REF. 1, p. 181)

48. A. Formaldehyde and formic acid are produced by oxidation of methyl alcohol. These substances are known to arrest retinal hexokinase activity. Impaired function of retinal hexokinase results in depression of glucose metabolism and a defect in the synthesis of ATP. (REF. 1, pp. 449–450)

49. A. Carbon monoxide is a colorless, odorless, and a nonirritating gas and because of this it is especially hazardous. It causes confusion and lethargy, which render the patient incapable of removing himself from the site of exposure. (REF. 1, p. 450)

50. E. The combination of the last two features is clinically designated as bronze diabetes. Additional characteristics of the usual case are increased body iron stores up to 80 g, elevated plasma iron up to 200–250 µg/100 ml, and excessive saturation of transferrin up to 60%–70%. (REF. 1, pp. 924–928)

51. E. The SER is rich in a wide variety of enzymes and is most abundant in those cells involved in the synthesis of lipids, particularly triglycerides, lipoprotein complexes, and steroids. One other function is that of glycogenolysis. In striated muscle the ER is called sarcoplasmic reticulum, which is thought to be involved in the conduction of contractile impulses from the surface membrane of the cell into the recesses of the muscle cell filled with myofilaments. (REF. 1, p. 27)

52. E. Anaphylatoxins effect the release of vasoactive compounds (i.e., histamine), which induce increased vascular permeability and smooth muscle contraction. Cell membrane damage may lead to cytolysis. (REF. 1, p. 166)

53. C. The first item describes hyaline perisplenitis which is not associated with any clinical dysfunction. Number 3 describes congestive splenomegaly and the nodules are called Gandy-Gamna nodules which are organized hemorrhages containing iron and calcium salts. Numbers 2 and 4 describe "sago" spleen and "lardaceous" spleen, respectively. (REF. 1, pp. 203–204)

54. E. It is not unusual to have a shrunken kidney even in the absence of intercurrent infection. This contraction is due to vascular narrowing induced by the deposition of amyloid within arterial and arteriolar walls. (REF. 1, p. 202)

55. C. Renal cell carcinoma invades the branches of the renal vein, extends to the main vein, then proceeds up to the inferior vena cava, sometimes reaching the right side of the heart. Hepatocarcinomas often penetrate portal and hepatic vein radicles to grow within the main venous channels. (REF. 1, p. 227)

56. A. Calcium ions provide the anionic bond between exposed negative charges of adjacent cell membranes. The architectural integrity of the epithelium is maintained by the intercellular junctions. (REF. 1, pp. 235–236)

57. A. The growth and size of fibroadenoma and uterine leiomyoma are estrogen-dependent. The growth of prostatic carcinoma can be inhibited by estrogen. (REF. 1, pp. 1136, 1175)

58. C. The central portion of the neoplasm is farthest from the blood supply; thus it undergoes ischemic necrosis when the tumor outgrows its blood supply. Atrophy of the surrounding normal parenchyma leaves the more resistant fibrous stroma of the normal tissue, which envelops the tumor mass, with the component elaborated by the neoplastic stroma. (REF. 1, pp. 223–225)

59. B. Both the cardiac and skeletal muscles are most capable of hypertrophy perhaps because they do not adapt to increased metabolic demands by mitotic division and the formation of more cells to share the work. (REF. 1, pp. 31–32)

60. E. In certain forms of glomerular disease, excessive leakage of proteins into the urine and reabsorption of lipoproteins by tubular cells lead to fat accumulation. Scavenger macrophages, whenever in contact with lipid debris or necrotic cells, may become stacked with neutral fats because of their phagocytic activities. Intracellular accumulation of cholesterol and cholesterol esters is encountered in a variety of diseases associated with hypercholesterolemia. The most important disorder is atherosclerosis in which ballooned-out myointimal cells within the intimal layer of the aorta and artery develop as a result of lipid accumulation. When these intracellular accumulations of cholesterol and cholesterol esters are found in the subepithelial connective tissue of the skin and in tendons they are referred to as xanthomas. (REF. 1, pp. 18–20)

61. B. Excesses of protein sufficient to cause a morphologically visible alteration are encountered only in renal epithelial cells of the proximal convoluted tubules and in plasma cells. The former is seen in the nephrotic syndrome that is characterized by heavy proteinuria owing to abnormal glomerular permeability. The reabsorption of the urinary proteins represents the basis of intracellular excess. Plasma cells engaged in active synthesis of immunoglobulin may become overloaded with this synthetic product to produce homogenous acidophilic large inclusions, the so-called Russell's bodies. (REF. 1, p. 21)

62. C. Except for lipofuscin and melanin, all the endogenous pigments are derived from hemoglobin. Melanin is an endogenous, brown-black pigment synthesized from tyrosine in melanocytes. Hemosiderin, an iron-storage substance, is a golden yellow-to-brown granular or crystalline pigment. Hemosiderin granules result from the aggregation of ferritin micelles. Hematin is of uncertain composition, is golden brown granular pigment and is virtually confined to RE cells. (REF. 1, pp. 23–25)

63. C. An acquired deficit in the cell-mediated response is encountered principally in Hodgkin's and sarcoidosis. This deficit may be accompanied by some diminished effectiveness of the humoral system. (REF. 1, pp. 172–173, 674)

64. E. The first three are examples of cellular and tissue injury mediated by humoral antibodies, whereas tuberculin reaction is principally a model of cell-mediated tissue injury. (REF. 1, p. 164)

65. B. Physiologic hyperplasia occurs in the gravid uterus and is accompanied by striking hypertrophy of preexisting smooth cells. The enlargement of one kidney when the other is destroyed or removed involves hypertrophy of individual nephrons produced by hyperplasia of tubular epithelial cells. The main process in 2 and 4 is hypertrophy without accompanying hyperplasia. (REF. 1, pp. 32–33)

66. E. Bactericidal and hemagglutinating antibodies are formed 7 to 10 days after meningococcal colonization of the upper respiratory mucosa. These antibodies, however, do not eliminate the carrier state but do impart a group-specific immunity. Carrier state is not uncommon, but a direct correlation between carrier rates and disease incidence has not been established. In a few cases, the disease results shortly after colonization, most frequently in the form of meningitis and meningococcemia. (REF. 3, p. 1088)

67. E. The diagnosis of syphilis must be suspected when a disseminated rash develops in a patient who appears to be "healthy." The skin lesions of the other bacteremic states are almost always accompanied by chills, malaise, and even prostration. (REF. 1, pp. 336–337)

68. E. The diagnosis of heterophile-negative infectious mononucleosis may be confirmed by an assay of EBV antibody. (REF. 3, pp. 715–716)

69. E. If caseation does not develop in the tuberculous lesion, the hard tubercle may be completely indistinguishable from other granulomatous lesions. Diagnosis of tuberculosis should not be made unless the acid-fast tubercle bacilli have been unmistakably identified in tissue sections or have been cultured from sputum, gastric washings, or tuberculous lesions. (REF. 1, pp. 64–65)

70. C. *L. monocytogenes* is a motile, nonsporulating, nonencapsulated gram-positive rod. On sheep blood agar it produces beta-hemolytic colonies. (REFS. 1, p. 328; 3, pp. 1093–1094)

71. C. Clinically, rat-bite fever is a relapsing fever. (REF. 1, p. 334)

72. B. Q fever may also cause vegetative endocarditis of mitral and aortic valves. (REF. 1, pp. 299–300)

73. D. This is a chlamydial infection. The diagnosis may be confirmed by the Frei skin test. (REF. 1, p. 291)

74. C. In a few cases the disease has been associated with injury by splinters and thorns. The lymph nodes show granulomatous abscess formation. (REF. 1, p. 291)

75. E. The cerebral involvement in *E. histolytica* infection should be distinguished from the primary amebic meningoencephalitis caused by *Acanthamoeba castellani*. (REF. 1, pp. 363–364)

76. E. Such fungal diseases may occur also in patients receiving antibiotics and corticosteroids or in patients with avitaminosis and severe malnutrition. (REF. 1, pp. 351–352)

77. D. The bubonic pattern of plague is the most common variant. (REF. 1, pp. 310–311)

78. C. Zenker's hyaline degeneration, or necrosis, may also be seen in the myocardium in severe diphtheria. (REF. 1, p. 1307; REF. 2, p. 306)

79. A. Legionella organisms are transmitted by the respiratory route. The organisms, which may exist for years in water reservoirs and air-conditioning systems containing blue-green algae, are fastidious to culture. In addition to immunofluorescence, they may be visualized by the Dierterle silver stain. (REF. 1, pp. 313–314)

80. E. Latent infections of cytomegalic inclusion disease (CID) can be demonstrated in the white blood cells of 5% of blood donors. CID can also be transmitted through breast milk, during passage of the fetus through the birth canal of a mother with latent infection, and by respiratory droplets. (REF. 1, p. 286)

81. C. Physiologic hyperplasia is best seen in number 2. Following every normal menstrual period, there is a rapid burst of proliferative activity, which might be considered as reparative proliferation or physiologic hyperplasia of the endometrium. One and 3 represent instances of excessive hormonal stimulation of target cells and are considered pathologic hyperplasia. (REF. 1, p. 32)

82. A. Dysplasia is an alteration in mature cells characterized by alteration in their size, shape, and organization. It is a controversial term in pathology, used both loosely and commonly. Strictly speaking, dysplasia means deranged development and is not an adaptive process. (REF. 1, pp. 34–35)

83. E. Hypoxic injury may be caused by loss of blood supply, as seen in blockage of arterial supply or venous drainage; loss of oxygen-carrying capacity of the blood seen in carbon monoxide poisoning and anemia; or poisoning of the oxidative enzymes within the cells as seen in cyanide poisoning. In carbon monoxide poisoning, carbon monoxyhemoglobin is formed and blocks the normal oxygen transport of oxyhemoglobin. Cytochrome oxidase is inactivated by cyanide. All of these adverse influences ultimately affect cellular aerobic respiration, oxidative phosphorylation, and synthesis of the high-energy bonds of ATP. (REF. 1, p. 4)

84. A. Prostaglandins, derived from arachidonic acid by the cyclooxygenase metabolic pathway, act predominantly as vasodilators thereby potentiating the edema of the acute inflammatory process. PGD_2 and PGF_2 also act as vasodilators. Bradykinin and histamine not only cause arteriolar vasodilatation but also increased permeability of venules. The potency of leukotriene in vascular permeability greatly exceeds that of histamine. (REF. 6, pp. 38–41)

85. A. Although a deficiency of lysyl oxidase causes a Marfan-like syndrome in animals, a similar deficiency is not known to occur in humans. It has been postulated that Marfan's syndrome may be the result of mutation of several genes involved in the synthesis of collagen or elastin. (REF. 6, p. 105)

86. A. The most common type of Down's syndrome, occurring in more than 90% of patients, is trisomy 21, usually the result of meiotic nondysjunction. About 4% of patients reveal translocation of the long arm of chromosome 21 to chromosome 22 or 14, while mosaicism consisting of a mixture of cells with 46 and 47 chromosomes occurs in another 2%. (REF. 6, pp. 121–122)

87. E. Human immunodeficiency virus (HIV) is T-lymphotropic, particularly for helper T cells of the subset OKT4. The T4/T8 ratio, usually about 2, decreases to about 0.5 in patients with ARC and AIDS. The destruction of T cells by the virus is manifested by disturbances of a variety of in vitro and in vivo T-cell functions such as susceptibility to neoplasms and opportunistic infections. (REF. 6, pp. 175–179)

88. E. In addition to the genes gag, pol, and env, which respectively encode the core protein, reverse transcriptase, and envelope proteins, HIV possesses five other genes which confer the unique characteristics and the unusual pathogenicity of the virus. (REF. 4, pp. 533–535)

89. E. The commonest metaplastic change involves the substitution of squamous for columnar, pseudostratified, glandular, or urothelial epithelium. Metaplasia may also occur in connective tissue, the usual form being osseous replacement of fibrous scars. (REF. 6, p. 185)

90. B. While renal cell carcinoma commonly invades the renal vein and inferior vena cava, hepatocellular carcinoma has a tendency to invade portal and hepatic veins. Breast and colonic carcinomas characteristically spread by lymphatic permeation. (REF. 6, p. 195)

91. A. (REF. 3, pp. 643–644, 824)

92. C. (REF. 1, pp. 653, 698)

93. B. (REF. 1, pp. 653, 698)

94. C. (REF. 1, pp. 158–159)

95. A. (REF. 1, p. 696)

96. C. (REF. 1, p. 163)

97. D. (REF. 1, p. 166)

98. B. (REF. 1, p. 166)

99. A. (REF. 1, pp. 169–170)

100. D. (REF. 1, pp. 169–170)

101. C. (REF. 1, p. 163)

102. A. (REF. 1, pp. 169–170)

103. D. Microorganisms coated with C3b, a component of the complement system generated by the classic or the alternate pathway, are more easily ingested by neutrophils and macrophages, which bear on their surface receptors for C3b and the Fc portion of the immunoglobulin molecule. (REF. 6, pp. 33, 39)

104. E. Interleukin-1, one of numerous biologically active products of macrophages, also activates T- and B-lymphocyte production and stimulates production of acute phase reactants by hepatocytes as well as collagenase by fibroblasts. (REF. 6, p. 43)

105. A. In Chediak-Higashi syndrome, an autosomal recessive disease, there is a defect in chemotaxis characterized by abnormalities of microtubules with subsequent impairment in the locomotion of leukocytes. (REF. 6, p. 36)

106. C. Sustained arteriolar vasodilation and potentiation of edema in acute inflammation is mediated by histamine, bradykinin, and prostaglandins PGI_2, PGE_2, PGD_2, and PGF_{2alpha}. Additionally, PGI_2 (protacyclin) inhibits platelet aggregation. (REF. 6, pp. 39 – 40)

107. B. Leukotrienes, products of arachidonic acid through the lipooxygenase pathway, actively participates in the acute inflammatory process. Whereas leukotrienes C_4 and D_4 increase vascular permeability, leukotriene B_4 is a powerful chemotactic agent for neutrophils and macrophages; it also contributes significantly to the process of margination. (REF. 6, pp. 39–40)

108. A. Postulated to be the major mechanism for microbicidal activity in neutrophils, the H_2O_2-halide-myeloperoxidase system, commences with the activation of NADH oxidase resulting in the production of superoxide anion and H_2O_2. The latter reacts with halide ions forming effective and powerful antimicrobial agents. (REF. 6, pp. 35–36)

109. B. See explanatory answer 107.

110. E. Diabetes mellitus is the most common predisposing factor of zygomycosis. The triad of diabetic acidosis, ophthalmoplegia, and signs of diffuse cerebral vascular disease is virtually diagnostic. The susceptible individual acquires the disease through inhalation of the spores either into the nasal passages or into the lungs. Cerebral zygomycosis usually occurs as a direct extension of nasal, sinus, or orbital disease. (REF. 1, p. 354)

111. D. The classic method of infection with *Sporothrix schenckii* is through a penetrating wound of the skin with a spore-bearing splinter or thorn. The rose gardener is highly vulnerable; the alcoholic gardener is extremely susceptible because of peripheral neuropathy. A slow-to-heal ulcer of the finger or hand appears 1–2 weeks following trauma. Because the fungus spreads up the lymphatics, a series of subcutaneous nodules form, become fixed to the skin, undergo necrosis, and eventually form secondary chancroid ulcers. These lesions are associated with lymphadenopathy. (REF. 3, p. 1157)

112. D. See explanatory answer 111. (REF. 3, pp. 1157–1158)

113. B. *Cryptococcus neoformans* characteristically does not elicit a cellular inflammatory response, even in immunocompetent individuals. This inert response together with the production of abundant polysaccharide capsular substance may lead to a misdiagnosis of mucin-producing carcinoma. The thick capsule surrounding a small spherical or single-budding (bud attached by constricted neck) yeast cell is mucicarmine-positive. This stain is virtually specific for the capsular material of *C. neoformans* and is specially helpful when its nonbudding yeast forms approach the size of *Blastomyces dermatidis*. (REF. 1, p. 355)

114. C. Sixty percent of infected individuals are asymptomatic; the rest develop influenzalike symptoms. Two percent of infected individuals present with residual cavitary or solid "coin" lesions of lungs; the cavitary lesions may simulate tuberculosis and solid lesions cannot be distinguished radiographically from a solitary primary or secondary neoplasm. Thick-walled spherules measuring >20 μ in diameter and containing numerous nonbudding endospores are virtually diagnostic of *C. immitis.* (REF. 1, pp. 357–358)

115. B. See explanatory answer 114. (REF. 1, p. 355)

116. C. See explanatory answer 114. (REF. 1, pp. 357–358)

117. A. Nails infected by dermatophytes have a chalky crumbling consistency and project above a thickened nail bed of keratinized epithelium and debris. *T. mentagrophytes* and *T. rubrum* are the most common causes. (REF. 3, p. 1159)

118. C. This may be used also for the isolation of *Neisseria meningitidis.* (REF. 3, p. 1357)

119. D. Chlamydospores are thick-walled and resistant spores that are produced by the rounding up and enlargement of the terminal cells of the hyphae. (REF. 1, pp. 1203, 1356)

120. A. This medium contains infusion from potatoes, sodium chloride, agar, and blood (human, rabbit, or sheep). It is used for the cultivation of *Bordetella pertussis.* (REF. 3, p. 1109)

121. B. Tellurite solution may be used to test the ability of certain mycobacterium of Runyon group III nonphotochromogens to reduce the tellurite rapidly to the black metallic tellurium. (REF. 3, p. 1091)

122. E. This method for identification of Cryptococcus is essential to the quick diagnosis and institution of immediate therapy, especially in cryptococcal meningitis. (REF. 1, p. 355)

123. D. This medium is used for the isolation of fungi when other contaminating microorganisms may be present. (REF. 3, pp. 1185–1186)

124. F. Infection by *Histoplasma capsulatum* occurs as primary pulmonary or disseminated histoplasmosis and rarely as sclerosing mediastinitis. Pathologic changes consisting of necrotizing epithelioid granulomata are found most commonly in the lungs, reticuloendothelial organs (lymph nodes, spleen, bone marrow, liver), and meninges. (REF. 1, p. 358)

125. B. Inhalation of infective material is the usual mode of transmission of *Cryptococcus neoformans*, a fungus excreted by birds, especially pigeons. The lung and the CNS are the most commonly affected organs. Pathologic changes range from virtually no inflammatory reaction to suppuration and fully formed granulomas. (REF. 1, p. 355)

126. A. Three distinct modes of tissue involvement by *Aspergillus* spp. are known: allergic, colonizing, and invasive. The growth of the fungus in cavities within the lung constitutes the colonizing type. In the invasive type, which occurs commonly in the immune suppressed patient, there is widespread hematogenous dissemination. (REF. 1, pp. 354–355)

127. G. Mucormycosis is caused by fungi from the *Rhizopus*, *Mucor*, and *Absidia* genera. The fungus has a tendency to invade blood vessels causing hematogenous dissemination. (REF. 1, p. 354)

128. C. Cryptosporidium infection of the gut is usually seen in immunosuppressed patients, especially those with the acquired immunodeficiency syndrome (AIDS). The disease is diagnosed by biopsy. (REF. 1, p. 365)

129. A. Marasmus is basically a state of starvation; the ratio of proteins to calories is usually normal. (REF. 1, p. 400)

130. C. The fatty change though seen in both disorders is more characteristic of kwashiorkor. It is due to decreased synthesis of lipoproteins necessary for the mobilization of fat from the liver. The fatty liver does not progress to cirrhosis. (REF. 1, p. 402)

131. B. This is associated with reduced number of circulating T cells which in part explains the high incidence of viral and fungal infections in these patients. (REF. 1, p. 407)

132. B. The skin lesions, which are pathognomonic, consist of areas of depigmentation and hyperpigmentation and in white children, patches of dusky erythema—"crazy pavement" appearance. (REF. 1, p. 401)

133. C. The anemia may also be polymorphic with signs of iron and/or folate deficiency in both peripheral smears and bone marrow. (REF. 1, p. 402)

134. D. Of the nutritional deficiency disorders, peripheral neuropathy is most frequently associated with deficiency of vitamin B, particularly thiamine. (REF. 1, p. 413)

135. A. A unique feature of RNA oncogenic virus is the occurrence of RNA-directed DNA polymerase (reverse transcriptase), which permits the transcription of viral DNA into virus-specific DNA. (REF. 6, p. 204; REF. 4, p. 527)

136. B. Five families of DNA oncogenic viruses exist: papoviruses, to which the human and animal papilloma viruses belong; adenoviruses of human and animal origin; herpes viruses to which Eptein-Barr virus and cytomegalovirus belong; hepadnavirus (human hepatitis); and poxviruses (*Molluscum contagiosum*). (REF. 4, p. 525)

137. C. There are two basic mechanisms by which oncogenic viruses induce transformation of host's cells: (1) incorporation of viral genome into the host's genome with the formation of a "transforming gene" or (2) induction of the expression of preexisting cellular gene. Specifically, oncogenic RNA viruses may cause cancer by inducing mutation of c-oncogenes by causing overexpression of c-oncogenes, or by inactivation of cellular regulatory genes. (REF. 6, p. 204; REF. 4, p. 521)

138. A. V-oncogenes are found in retroviruses and they account for the transforming property of some of these viruses. (REF. 6, p. 205)

139. A. Human T-lymphotropic virus (HTLV) has a propensity for T-lymphocytes. HTLV-1 has been isolated from patients with adult T-cell leukemia, a disease which is clustered in southern Japan, the Caribbean basin and the southern United States. The virus, which belongs to the C-type RNA oncogenic viruses, is exogenous, i.e., the viral genetic information is not a constant part of the genetic constitution of the human lymphocytes. (REF. 4, p. 205; REF. 4, pp. 529–531)

140. B. The inability of cells transformed by DNA oncogenic viruses to replicate is one of the properties that distinguishes RNA from DNA tumor viruses. (REF. 6, p. 205)

141. D. Proto- or cellular oncogenes, close relatives of v-oncogenes, are present in normal cells of diverse organisms in the animal kingdom. It has been postulated that they are essential to normal cellular function. They may, however, be activated and converted to cancer genes. Many mechanisms by which this transformation occurs have been proposed. (REF. 6, pp. 523–524)

2 Cardiovascular System

---

142. Which of the following most accurately describes the events that lead to the characteristic features of paradoxic myocardial infarction?
    A. Atherosclerosis with thrombosis of intramyocardial arteries
    B. Severe stenosis of right coronary artery with infarction of an area supplied by left anterior descending artery
    C. Acute myocardial infarction without demonstrable occlusion of coronary arteries
    D. Acute infarction that involves the entire myocardium from the pericardium to the endocardium (transmural infarction)
    E. Acute myocardial infarction due to coronary arteritis rather than atherosclerosis

143. Patent ductus arteriosus shows all of the following features EXCEPT
   A. it is an integral lesion of the tetralogy of Fallot
   B. it has a striking female preponderance
   C. right ventricular hypertrophy
   D. development of cyanosis is in the late stages
   E. a continuous systolic and diastolic murmur

144. The most specific parameter in the enzymatic diagnosis of acute myocardial infarction is the serum activity of
   A. total lactic acid dehydrogenase (LDH)
   B. total creatine phosphokinase (CPK)
   C. serum glutamic oxaloacetic transaminase (GOT)
   D. CPK-MB isoenzyme
   E. LDH5 isoenzyme

145. Which of the following shows an inverse relationship to the risk for developing atherosclerosis?
   A. High-density lipoprotein
   B. Low-density lipoprotein
   C. Very-low-density lipoprotein
   D. Cholesterol
   E. Triglycerides

146. Monckeberg's arteriosclerosis is characterized by all of the following EXCEPT
   A. medial calcification
   B. involvement of predominantly small-to-medium-sized muscular arteries
   C. luminal narrowing with consequent ischemic changes
   D. rarity in persons younger than 50 years of age
   E. a distinct entity from atherosclerosis

147. The involvement of the aortic arch by an inflammatory lesion composed of adventitial mononuclear infiltrate, perivascular cuffing of vasa vasorum, and acute and/or chronic inflammation of the media is characteristic of
    A. thromboangiitis obliterans
    B. syphilitic aortitis
    C. infectious aortitis
    D. rheumatoid aortitis
    E. Takayasu's arteritis

148. All of the following may usually be found in uncomplicated right-sided heart failure EXCEPT
    A. subcutaneous edema of dependent parts of the body
    B. hydrothorax
    C. passive congestion of the spleen
    D. pulmonary edema
    E. visceral venous congestion

149. High-output cardiac failure is NOT found in
    A. hyperthyroidism
    B. Paget's disease of bone
    C. severe anemia
    D. myocardial infarction
    E. thiamine deficiency

150. Fatty change with "tigroid" appearance in the myocardium is characteristic of
    A. alcoholic cardiac injury
    B. diabetes mellitus
    C. chronic anemia
    D. hyperthyroidism
    E. obesity

151. MacCallum's patch is usually located in the
    A. right atrium
    B. left atrium
    C. right ventricle
    D. left ventricle
    E. pericardium

152. According to prevalent opinion, a typical Aschoff nodule does NOT include
    A. Anitschkow's cells
    B. multinucleated histiocytic giant cells
    C. multinucleated myogenic giant cells
    D. fibrinoid necrosis
    E. fibroblasts

153. Which part of the aorta is least severely affected by atherosclerosis?
    A. Abdominal aorta
    B. Root of the aorta
    C. Branching points of the vessels originating from the aorta
    D. Arch of the aorta
    E. Thoracic aorta

154. Mitral valve prolapse is not characterized by which of the following?
    A. The posterior valve leaflet is always involved
    B. Clinically manifests as a mid-systolic click with or without a holosystolic murmur
    C. Causes moderate-to-severe mitral stenosis
    D. Sections of the affected leaflets show myxomatous degeneration
    E. Is a condition occurring more commonly in young women

155. Which of the following most accurately describes the typical valvular vegetation of acute rheumatic carditis?
    A. Small 1- to 2-mm verrucae along the lines of closure of the valve leaflets
    B. Friable irregular vegetations along the free margins of the valve leaflets
    C. Small masses of fibrin and other blood elements located on the free edge of valve leaflets
    D. Warty excrescences which may occur singly or multiply in a random fashion anywhere on the valve leaflets
    E. Small vegetations located behind the cusps of the valves

156. A myocarditis that histologically reveals focal myocardial necrosis, lymphocytes, eosinophils, plasma cells, macrophages, and multinucleated giant cells is most likely to be
   A. Chagas' disease
   B. Fiedler's myocarditis
   C. trichinosis
   D. cytomegalovirus myocarditis
   E. myocarditis complicating systemic lupus erythematosus

157. An aneurysm derived from arterio-venous communication may be termed
   A. cirsoid (racemose)
   B. mycotic
   C. false
   D. berry
   E. dissecting

DIRECTIONS: For each of the questions or incomplete statements below, **one** or **more** of the answers or completions given is correct. Select
   A   if only *1, 2, and 3* are correct
   B   if only *1 and 3* are correct
   C   if only *2 and 4* are correct
   D   if only *4* is correct
   E   if all are correct

---

158. The essential component(s) of the atherosclerotic lesion is (are)
   1. lipid deposition
   2. smooth muscle proliferation
   3. accumulation of connective tissue fibers and matrix
   4. chronic inflammatory cells

Directions Summarized				
A	B	C	D	E
1,2,3	1,3	2,4	4	All are
only	only	only	only	correct

159. Infective endocarditis in the drug addict is characterized by which of the following?
    1. The tricuspid valve is involved in more than 50% of cases
    2. *Candida* endocarditis is more common in this group of patients when compared with the general population
    3. Most addicts with endocarditis have no preexisting valvular disease
    4. *Staphylococcus aureus* is isolated most commonly

160. In hypertrophic cardiomyopathy (CMP)
    1. there is a disproportionate thickening of the interventricular septum
    2. the ventricular cavities are often dilated
    3. distinctive microscopic changes consisting of myocardial fiber disarray are usually found
    4. intraventricular thrombosis is common

161. A strong relationship exists between malignant tumors and which of the following?
    1. Phlegmasia alba dolens
    2. Migratory thrombophlebitis
    3. Phlebothrombosis
    4. Superior vena cava syndrome

162. The prognosis of tetralogy of Fallot is worse than that of Eisenmenger's complex primarily due to
    1. hypertrophy of right ventricle
    2. dextroposition of large vessels
    3. ventricular septal defect
    4. prepulmonic valvular stenosis

163. Available evidence points to an immunologic mechanism in which of the following cardiomyopathies?
    1. Rheumatoid arthritis
    2. Rheumatic fever
    3. Systemic lupus erythematosus
    4. Endomyocardial fibrosis

164. Myocardial contraction bands
    1. have been described around the margins of acute myocardial infarction
    2. are synonymous with wavy myocardial fibers
    3. may be seen in patients undergoing coronary artery bypass surgery
    4. are found only in enlarged hearts

165. In a patient with significantly narrowed coronary arteries, acute myocardial infarction is caused by
    1. increased myocardial demand
    2. diminished availability of oxygen in the blood
    3. coronary spasm
    4. reduced coronary arterial flow

166. Which of the following statements is (are) true regarding the origin and the role of smooth muscles in the pathogenesis of the atheromatous plaque?
    1. The smooth muscle cells are derived, in part, from cells which migrate from the media
    2. Growth factors derived from platelets and macrophages may be responsible for stimulating proliferation of smooth muscle cells
    3. Some of the foam cells seen in atheromatous plaques are derived from smooth muscle cells
    4. Smooth muscle cells elaborate collagen, elastic tissue, and proteoglycans

Directions Summarized				
A	B	C	D	E
1,2,3	1,3	2,4	4	All are
only	only	only	only	correct

167. Which of these changes would be expected to occur in a myocardial infarct 12 hours old?
    1. Reduced myocardial level of succinic dehydrogenase (SDH)
    2. Electron microscopic demonstration of mitochondrial swelling and distortion of cristae
    3. Wavy myocardial fibers at the border of the infarct
    4. Heavy polymorphonuclear leucocytic infiltrate

168. The beneficial (protective) effects of strenuous exercise against the development of myocardial infarction is due to
    1. augmentation of fibrinolytic response
    2. elevation of the level of serum high-density lipo-proteins
    3. hereditary and constitutional factors
    4. strong psychological effect, which tends to lower the blood pressure

169. Which of the following is (are) true for unstable angina pectoris?
    1. Coronary spasm has been implicated as the etiology in some patients
    2. Patients may develop fatal arrhythmias
    3. Focal myocardial necrosis may be demonstrated
    4. It is synonymous with Prinzmetal's variant angina

DIRECTIONS: Each group of questions below consists of five lettered headings followed by a list of numbered words, phrases, or statements. For **each** numbered word, phrase, or statement, select the **one** lettered heading that is most closely associated with it. Each lettered heading may be selected once, more than once, or not at all.

Questions 170–176:
- A. Serous pericarditis
- B. Fibrinous pericarditis
- C. Suppurative pericarditis
- D. Constrictive pericarditis
- E. Hemorrhagic pericarditis

170. Pyogenic coccal infection

171. *Mycobacterium tuberculosis*

172. Azotemia

173. Metastatic neoplasm

174. Collagen diseases

175. Rheumatic fever

176. Myocardial infarction

Questions 177–183:
- A. Muscular arteries
- B. Small arteries and arterioles
- C. Arterioles and capillaries
- D. Capillaries, venules, and arterioles
- E. Arteries, veins, and nerves

177. Hypersensitivity angiitis

178. Systemic lupus erythematosus

179. Polyarteritis nodosa

180. Buerger's disease

181. Wegener's granulomatosis

182. Rheumatic arteritis

183. Rheumatoid arteritis

Questions 184–189:
- **A.** Infective endocarditis
- **B.** Nonbacterial verrucous endocarditis (Libman-Sacks)
- **C.** Nonbacterial thrombotic endocarditis
- **D.** Rheumatic endocarditis
- **E.** Fungal endocarditis

184. Flat, spreading on both surfaces of valve leaflets

185. Large and friable vegetations at closure margins

186. Commonly associated with malignant tumors

187. Vegetations along closure margins

188. Observed in acute systemic lupus erythematosus

189. Of controversial clinical significance

Answers and Comments

142. B. Paradoxic infarction results from the following sequence of events. Stenosis of left coronary artery results in development of collateral circulation from the right coronary artery. Subsequent stenosis and coronary occlusion of right coronary artery lead to infarction of the area supported by the collateral circulation. (REF. 1, p. 559)

143. A. The increased blood flow to the right heart also produces pulmonary hypertension, dilatation of pulmonary vascular tree, and pulmonary hypertension. (REF. 1, p. 588)

144. D. CPK-MB isoenzyme begins to appear very early in the course of an acute myocardial infarction, peaks within 24–48 hours, and then progressively declines. The serum level of CPK-MB may be used as a determinant of the extent of myocardial damage. (REF. 3, p. 276)

145. A. High-density lipoprotein, composed of high quantities of phospholipids and low in cholesterol, has been termed "protective molecule" because it is postulated that it facilitates the mobilization of cholesterol from smooth muscle cells. Low-density lipoprotein, on the other hand, contains about 70% of serum cholesterol and strongly correlates with the risk for atherosclerosis. (REF. 3, p. 196)

146. C. This disorder, of uncertain etiology, occurs equally in both sexes and is of relatively no clinical significance. It should be distinguished from atherosclerosis because of the clinical complications. (REF. 1, p. 518)

147. E. Takayasu's arteritis (aortic arch syndrome, pulseless disease) typically involves the aortic arch and, less commonly, other parts of the aorta. Macroscopically, the aorta is thickened and shows intimal wrinkling. The orifices of the major branches originating from the aortic arch may be narrowed or obliterated. In addition to the histologic features detailed in the question, granulomatous lesions may be found in the media. (REF. 1, p. 526)

148. D. In left-sided heart failure, the major manifestations are those associated with passive congestion and edema of the lungs. In more severe cases, pulmonary hypertension results, leading to failure of the right side of the heart. Although failure of the right side of the heart is usually combined with that of the left, there are instances of isolated right heart failure. (REF. 1, p. 550)

149. D. Acute cardiac failure is caused by such conditions as myocardial injury due to coronary occlusion, obstruction to cardiac outflow, as in massive pulmonary embolism or cardiac tamponade resulting from sudden hemopericardium incident to rupture of the heart. In acute failure, there is a sudden reduction or cessation of cardiac output. (REF. 2, p. 561)

150. C. Macroscopically, there are two forms of fatty degeneration: patchy and diffuse. The patchy form, also known as "tigroid," "tabby cat," and "thrush-breast" appearance, affects the subendocardial portion of the myocardium and the papillary muscles particularly in the left ventricle. Beneath the surface a mottling can be seen in forms of irregular yellowish streaks or lines of involved muscles alternating with lines of unaffected muscle, thus the descriptive nomenclature. (REF. 1, pp. 19–20)

151. B. The maplike thickenings of the mural endocardium in the left atrium in rheumatic heart disease are called MacCallum's plaques. These are thought to represent subendocardial aggregations of Aschoff bodies accompanied by pooling of ground substance. This may eventually undergo fibrosis leaving an irregular area of endocardial wrinkling. (REF. 1, p. 574)

152. C. The Aschoff nodules represent the distinctive proliferative phase of this disease. The central focus is surrounded by a rim of mononuclear white cells, fibroblasts, large modified fibroblasts, large modified mesenchymal cells known as Anitschkow's myocytes, and an occasional multinucleated Aschoff giant cell. The origin of these cells is controversial, but most investigators consider them to be altered fibroblasts rather than modified muscle cells. (REF. 1, p. 572)

153. B. In its severest form, atherosclerosis is complicated by calcification, thrombosis, hemorrhage, ulceration, and aneurysmal dilatation. (REF. 1, pp. 509–512)

154. C. Mitral valve prolapse is due to excessively large leaflet and/or elongated chordae tendinae. During the systole the valve leaflets balloon back into the left atrium. This condition may be complicated by calcification of the basal portion of the leaflets, infective endocarditis, or rupture of chordae tendineae. (REF. 1, pp. 576–577)

155. A. The vegetations of rheumatic carditis occur on the surfaces exposed to the forward flow of blood. They may also be found on the chordae tendineae. Histologic examination shows fibrinoid necrosis with nonspecific inflammation; occasionally, however, fibroblasts, Anitschkow cells, and Aschoff bodies may be found. (REF. 1, p. 573)

156. B. The etiology of Fiedler's myocarditis is unknown. The presence of plasma cells and eosinophils suggests a disease of immune origin. (REF. 1, pp. 595–596)

157. A. Mycotic aneurysms result from microbial infection of the walls of vessels; the wall of a false aneurysm is fibrous, being composed of adventitia and perivascular tissue. Berry aneurysms are small saccular vascular dilatation on the order of 0.5 to 2 cm and are most often encountered in cerebral vessels. Dissecting aneurysms refer to dissection within the vessel wall originating from an intimal tear. (REF. 2, p. 707; REF. 1, p. 300)

158. A. The components occur in varying proportions giving rise to several gross morphologic forms of atherosclerosis. The plaque may be complicated by calcification, ulceration, superimposed thrombosis, hemorrhage, and aneurysm formation. (REF. 1, pp. 509–511)

159. E. The most common etiologic agents of the infective endocarditis of the addict are those organisms that constitute the normal skin flora. *S. aureus* alone accounts for more than 50% of the attacks in addicts. (REF. 1, p. 581)

160. B. Hypertrophic CMP, also called asymmetrical septal hypertrophy, may occur in a sporadic or familial form, the latter being related to autosomal dominant transmission. The free left ventricle may be normal or hypertrophied but the most typical change is disproportionate septal hypertrophy. Additionally there may be plaquelike endocardial thickening of the left ventricular outflow tract. (REF. 1, pp. 597–599)

161. C. Phlegmasia alba dolens, usually occurring in women in the third trimester of pregnancy, consists of painful swelling of lower extremities. The disorder is a special type of phlebothrombosis of obscure etiology but probably results from a combination of thrombosis, perivenous inflammation, and lymphatic blockage. (REF. 1, p. 537)

162. D. Prepulmonic stenosis seen in tetralogy of Fallot usually produces a very serious defect in pulmonary circulation. Patients with Eisenmenger's complex usually have adequate pulmonary vascular flow and hence better prognosis. (REF. 1, p. 590)

163. A. The pathogenesis of endomyocardial fibrosis has not been elucidated. It is seen most frequently in Africa. No abnormalities in the serum complement levels or presence of abnormal proteins in the serum have been observed in association with this entity. (REF. 1, p. 599)

164. B. Contraction bands are eosinophilic bands that lie transversely in myocardial fibers, usually found at the periphery of acute myocardial infarcts. By electron microscopy, there is shortening of sarcomeres and approximation of I bands. (REF. 1, p. 561)

165. D. Coronary artery perfusion may also be reduced by hypotension, stenosing fibrocalcific disease of the aortic valve, and tricuspid regurgitation. Acute myocardial infarction may be precipitated in these instances in patients with a previous significant arterial narrowing. (REF. 1, pp. 553–555)

166. E. Foam cells comprising smooth muscle cells and macrophages contain cholesterol and cholesterol esters. (REF. 1, pp. 516–517)

167. A. In addition to SDH, the infarcted myocardium also shows a decreased level of glycogen (demonstrable by the PAS stain), cytochrome oxidase, and phosphorylase. By light microscopy, there is early coagulation necrosis, hemorrhage, and sparse neutrophilic exudate. (REF. 6, pp. 323–326)

168. A. There is no firm conclusion about the role of strenuous exercise such as jogging in protecting against myocardial infarction. Statistical data, however, show that the risk of heart attack is lower among people who engage in a regular exercise schedule or whose profession or job involves physical exertion. (REF. 6, p. 321)

169. A. Three forms of angina pectoris (AP) are defined: typical, Prinzmetal's, and unstable. Typical AP is related to exertion and increased oxygen demand by the myocardium. Prinzmetal's variant refers to AP occurring at rest most probably caused by coronary artery spasm or platelet aggregation resulting in transmural ischemia. In unstable AP, chest pain is more frequent and/or lasts for longer periods than that in typical AP. (REF. 6, p. 319)

170. C. (REF. 1, p. 603)

171. D. (REF. 1, p. 604)

172. B. (REF. 1, p. 603)

173. E. (REF. 1, p. 604)

174. A. (REF. 1, p. 603)

175. B. (REF. 1, p. 603)

176. B. (REF. 1, p. 603)

177. D. (REF. 1, p. 522)

178. C. (REF. 1, p. 183)

179. A. (REF. 1, p. 520)

180. E. (REF. 1, p. 526)

181. B. (REF. 1, p. 523)

182. C. (REF. 1, p. 574)

183. A. (REF. 1, p. 528)

184. B. (REF. 1, p. 187)

185. A. (REF. 1, p. 582)

186. C. (REF. 1, p. 584)

187. D. (REF. 1, p. 574)

188. B. (REF. 1, p. 187)

189. C. (REF. 1, p. 584)

3 Gastrointestinal System

DIRECTIONS: Each of the questions or incomplete statements below is followed by five suggested answers or completions. Select the **one** that is best in each case.

---

190. The mechanism of the pathogenesis of infective enterocolitis by which organism does *not* involve invasion of the gut?
    A. *Campylobacter jejuni*
    B. *Shigella sonnei*
    C. *Vibrio cholerae*
    D. *Entamoeba histolytica*
    E. *Mycobacterium tuberculosis*

191. All of the following are true of achalasia EXCEPT
    A. it may be caused by *Trypanosoma cruzi* infection
    B. there is partial or incomplete relaxation of lower esophageal sphincter (LES)
    C. dilatation and tortuosity of the esophagus about the level of the sphincter is the rule
    D. consistently shows the absence of myenteric ganglion cells in the lower sphincter
    E. the esophageal mucosa may show ulceroinflammatory and fibrotic lesions

192. All of the following mechanisms have been proposed for the pathogenesis of gastric stress ulcers due to extensive burns (Curling's ulcers) EXCEPT

A. hypersecretion of gastric acid
B. mucosal hypoxia related to neurogenic vasoconstriction
C. mucosal hypoxia related to catecholamine-induced vasoconstriction
D. systemic (metabolic) acidosis
E. lowering of intracellular pH levels

193. The most vulnerable part of the colon to transmural infarction (gangrene) caused by thrombotic or embolic occlusion of the celiac–mesenteric axis is the

A. splenic flexure
B. cecum
C. transverse colon
D. ascending colon
E. rectum

194. Which of the following is NOT true of the laceration in the Mallory-Weiss syndrome?

A. Linear configuration
B. Variable length—from a few millimeters to several centimeters
C. Usually observed in the distal esophagus
D. Aligned at right angle to the long axis of the esophagus
E. May stretch across the esophagogastric junction

195. Grossly, gastric carcinoma most frequently assumes which of the following morphologic patterns?

A. Diffusely infiltrative (linitis plastica)
B. Ulcerative, infiltrative
C. Fungating
D. Polypoid
E. Superficial spreading

196. Which of the following statements concerning carcinoid tumor is NOT true?
    A. The neoplasm arises from basigranular Kulchitsky's cells
    B. The neoplasm most frequently occurs in distal ileum
    C. Episodic skin flushing, diarrhea, bronchospasm, and hypotension are the symptoms of the carcinoid syndrome
    D. Involvement of the tricuspid valves is the usual cardiac lesion in cases where the heart is involved
    E. The most common site of metastases is the lung

197. In colonic mucosal biopsies, the presence of which of the following microscopic features favors the diagnosis of Crohn's colitis over ulcerative colitis?
    A. Crypt abscesses
    B. Intense submucosal inflammation with minimal mucosal involvement
    C. Mucosal atrophy
    D. Malalignment of mucosal crypts
    E. Loss of goblet cells

198. Which of the following features is characteristically associated with ulcerative colitis presenting as toxic megacolon?
    A. Pseudopolyps
    B. Extensive mucosal and submucosal fibrosis
    C. Metaplasia of Paneth's cell
    D. Evidence of vasculitis
    E. Muscular atrophy

199. Among the colorectal lesions of epithelial derivation the most frequently encountered lesion is
    A. adenomatous polyp
    B. villous polyp
    C. mixed adenomatous and villous polyp
    D. hyperplastic polyp
    E. adenocarcinoma

200. The incidence of carcinoma arising in polyps of colorectal region is highest in
  A. pure adenomatous polyps
  B. pure villous polyps
  C. hybrid adenomatous and villous polyps
  D. hyperplastic polyps
  E. pseudopolyps

201. Inflammatory reaction and/or lymphatic obstruction are the pathogenic mechanisms for the production of malabsorption in all of the following EXCEPT
  A. lymphoma
  B. Whipple's disease
  C. regional enteritis
  D. jejunal diverticulosis
  E. tuberculosis

202. Hemorrhoids are most frequently encountered in subjects with
  A. good general health
  B. alcoholic cirrhosis
  C. colorectal carcinoma
  D. portal vein thrombosis
  E. massive uterine leiomyoma

203. Among the carcinomas of the anal region, which of the following is the predominant histologic type?
  A. Mucoepidermoid carcinoma
  B. Colloid carcinoma
  C. Squamous cell carcinoma
  D. Basaloid carcinoma
  E. Adenoacanthoma

204. Malignant melanoma occurring in which of the following segments of the gastrointestinal tract is most likely to be a primary neoplasm?
  A. Stomach
  B. Duodenum
  C. Jejunum
  D. Colon
  E. Anal canal

205. In Zollinger-Ellison syndrome the diarrhea seems to be related to
- **A.** the effect of gastrin on intestinal motility
- **B.** the effect of gastrin on water absorption
- **C.** elaboration of vasoactive intestinal peptide
- **D.** excessive gastric acid production
- **E.** multiple jejunal ulcers

206. In which of the following disorders causing malabsorption syndrome may large pale histocytes containing PAS-positive inclusions be found?
- **A.** Amyloidosis
- **B.** Tangier's disease
- **C.** Nontropical sprue
- **D.** Whipple's disease
- **E.** Abetalipoproteinemia

207. Pseudomembrane formation typical of *Clostridium difficile* pseudomembranous colitis is most likely caused by
- **A.** direct toxic effect of a broad spectrum antibiotic such as cephalosporins
- **B.** simple overgrowth of a variety of other gram-negative bacteria
- **C.** invasiveness of *C. difficile*
- **D.** enterotoxin of *C. difficile*
- **E.** none of the above

DIRECTIONS: For each of the questions or incomplete statements below, **one** or **more** of the answers or completions given is correct. Select

- **A** if only *1, 2, and 3* are correct
- **B** if only *1 and 3* are correct
- **C** if only *2 and 4* are correct
- **D** if only *4* is correct
- **E** if all are correct

		Directions Summarized		
A	B	C	D	E
1,2,3	1,3	2,4	4	All are
only	only	only	only	correct

208. Histologic type(s) of malignant lymphoma that may occur in the gastrointestinal tract include(s)
1. small cell diffuse malignant lymphoma
2. Hodgkin's disease
3. large cell cleaved cell type malignant lymphoma
4. Burkitt's lymphoma

209. Which of the following (has) have been unequivocably associated with transmural infarction (gangrene) of the small intestines?
1. Severe atherosclerosis
2. Rheumatoid arthritis
3. Bacterial endocarditis
4. Fibromuscular hyperplasia of the intestinal arteries

210. The frequent complication(s) of ulcerative colitis include(s)
1. perforation
2. toxic megacolon
3. venous thrombosis
4. colonic carcinoma

211. In melanosis coli, the
1. pigment accumulates in mucosal cells of the colon
2. pigment is melaninlike
3. prognosis is similar to that of malignant melanoma
4. pigment is found almost exclusively in mononuclear cells of the lamina propria

212. Mesenteric thrombi of the arterial type are associated with
1. heart disease
2. embolism
3. atherosclerosis
4. upper abdominal surgery

213. Acinic cell tumor of the salivary gland typically
    1. arises from the minor salivary glands
    2. has been postulated to arise from serous acinar cells
    3. is a benign tumor with no malignant potential
    4. shows PAS-positive granules in the cytoplasm of tumor cells

214. Impairment of digestive function is the pathogenic mechanism for malabsorption in
    1. biliary cirrhosis
    2. massive bowel resection
    3. subtotal gastrectomy
    4. gastroileostomy

215. Which of the following salivary gland tumors has a prominent lymphoid component?
    1. Pleomorphic adenoma
    2. Cylindroma
    3. Acinic cell adenocarcinoma
    4. Warthin's tumor

216. Which of the following is (are) true of pneumatosis cystoides intestinalis?
    1. Gas-filled cysts are found in the intestinal mucosa and submucosa
    2. It may be associated with duodenal ulcer
    3. Spontaneous resolution of the lesion occurs
    4. It shows morphologic resemblance to cystosarcoma phyllodes of the breast

---

DIRECTIONS: The group of questions below consists of five lettered headings followed by a list of numbered words, phrases, or statements. For **each** numbered word, phrase, or statement, select the **one** lettered heading that is most closely associated with it. Each lettered heading may be selected once, more than once, or not at all.

Questions 217–223:
  A. Predominant involvement of small intestine
  B. Predominant involvement of colon
  C. Ileocecal area
  D. Both small intestine and colon equally affected
  E. None of the above

217. Actinomycosis

218. Typhoid

219. Bacillary dysentery

220. Potassium enteropathy

221. Familial multiple polyposis

222. Whipple's disease

223. Plummer-Vinson syndrome

DIRECTIONS: Each set of lettered headings below is followed by a list of numbered words or phrases. For each numbered word or phrase select

  A if the item is associated with (A) *only*
  B if the item is associated with (B) *only*
  C if the item is associated with *both* (A) *and* (B)
  D if the item is associated with *neither* (A) *nor* (B)

Questions 224–228:
  A. Chronic atrophic gastritis
  B. Chronic hypertrophic gastritis
  C. Both
  D. Neither

224. Antigastric parietal cell antibodies

225. "Intestinalization" of the mucosa

226. Associated with Zollinger-Ellison syndrome

227. Predisposition to benign peptic ulcer

228. Granulomatous inflammation

Questions 229–233:
   A. Celiac disease (nontropical sprue)
   B. Tropical sprue
   C. Both
   D. Neither

229. Long-term antibiotic administration may be therapeutic

230. Macrophages containing PAS-positive glycoprotein granules

231. Many patients have HLA-B8 phenotype

232. Electron-microscopic examination shows markedly shortened and distorted microvilli with abnormal mitochondrial structure

233. Steatorrhea, weight loss, anorexia, abdominal distention, and borborygmi

Answers and Comments

190. C. *Vibrio cholerae* and certain strains of *E. coli* activate the enzyme adenylate cyclase which in turn stimulates fluid and electrolyte secretion, the cause of diarrheal illness associated with infections by these organisms. Other enteroinvasive organisms include *Salmonella* and *Yersinia enterocolitis*. (REF. 1, pp. 833–834)

191. D. Achalasia also shows aperistalsis and increased basal tone of the lower esophageal sphincter. In general there is a loss of myenteric ganglion cells in the body of the esophagus; it is controversial whether the ganglion cells in the lower segment are normal, reduced, or absent. Achalasia may be complicated by esophageal cancer in 2% to 7% of patients. (REF. 1, p. 799)

192. A. Stress ulcers of the stomach are generally associated with normal to low levels of gastric acid. However, in Cushing's ulcer, increased intracranial pressure directly stimulated vagal nuclei leading to gastric acid hypersecretion. (REF. 1, p. 813)

193. A. The splenic flexure is the watershed between the areas supplied by the superior and inferior mesenteric arteries, hence, the vulnerability of this portion of the colon. (REF. 1, p. 832)

194. D. The esophageal laceration in Mallory-Weiss syndrome is almost always aligned parallel to the long axis of the esophagus. (REF. 1, p. 800)

195. B. Grossly, gastric carcinoma generally assumes one of the two principal patterns of growth: massive intraluminal mass formation, or invasive-infiltrative growth. The gross appearance of the lesion may be altered by secondary surface erosions and, less commonly, from a multicentric origin. Ulcerative-infiltrative neoplasms, the most frequent, account for 30%–40% of all gastric carcinomas. (REF. 1, pp. 822–823)

196. E. By and large, carcinoid tumor occurs in the gastrointestinal tract with the distal ileum as the primary site. The regional lymph nodes and the liver are the common sites for metastases. (REF. 1, p. 843)

197. B. Fundamentally, Crohn's colitis can be regarded as the disease of the submucosa; ulcerative colitis, by contrast, primarily is the disease of mucosa. Mucosal atrophy, malalignments of mucosal crypts, and depletion of goblet cells are changes characteristically observed in ulcerative colitis. (REF. 1, pp. 838–840)

198. D. Evidence of acute vasculitis is frequently observed during the toxic megacolon phase of ulcerative colitis. The other morphologic features mentioned in the choices are primarily the features of indolent disease. Pseudopolyps form as a result of repair "overshooting the mark." Fibrosis represents severe antecedent injury with necrosis. Profuse bleeding and associated fluid and electrolyte disturbances in toxic megacolon may prove life-threatening. Perforation and peritonitis are other serious complications of this form of ulcerative colitis. (REF. 1, p. 860)

199. D. Hyperplastic polyps of colorectal mucosa are "dewdrop"-like knobs and represent areas of differentiated glandular hyperplasia. Generally measuring 3 mm or less in diameter, these polyps account for about 90% of all polypoid lesions and they lack the attributes of neoplasia, do not have any proclivity for malignant change, and appear inconsequential in the genesis of colorectal carcinoma. (REF. 1, p. 864)

200. B. Villous adenoma has been widely regarded as a forerunner of colorectal carcinoma. The genesis of invasive carcinoma in this neoplasm has been variously estimated to occur in 30%–70% of the lesions. The lack of agreement on the data reported in the literature can be attributed largely to the inconsistent use of terms and definitions and variable extent of the histologic study. In one large study, carcinoma was observed in 48% of villous adenomas, 18% of hybrid adenomatous and papillary lesions, and in 1% of adenomatous polyps. (REF. 1, p. 866)

201. D. The pathogenetic mechanism involved in the production of malabsorption syndrome in jejunal diverticulosis is believed to be the "blind loop syndrome" with associated changes in the intestinal bacterial flora. In the other disease processes included in the stem of this question, lymphatic obstruction and stasis interfere with the absorptive function of the gut, leading to malabsorption. (REF. 1, p. 846)

202. A. The hemorrhoids, varicosities of the anorectal region that develop in patients with cirrhosis and portal vein thrombosis, reflect the development of collateral anastomotic channels between the tributaries of the inferior and superior hemorrhoidal plexus. The development of hemorrhoids in association with massive uterine leiomyomata and other pelvic neoplasms is secondary to external pressure and, in the case of rectal carcinoma, constipation and associated straining at the time of defecation. (REF. 1, p. 858)

203. C. The predominant histologic variant of carcinoma of the anal region is epidermoid carcinoma arising from the squamous epithelium of the anal canal. The distant spread generally occurs by way of the right perianal lymphatic plexuses to the lymph nodes in the inguinal regions. The basaloid tumors have been thought to carry a more favorable prognosis than the epidermoid variants. The mucoepidermoid carcinoma, anal duct carcinoma, and the adenoacanthomas of anal region are rare neoplasms. (REF. 1, p. 1086)

204. E. Among the malignant melanomas encountered in the various parts of the gastrointestinal tract, only those observed in the esophagus and the anal canal are generally considered to be primary neoplasms. In these locations, the primary nature of malignant melanoma can often be proved by demonstration of junctional change. In other parts of the gastrointestinal tract, melanomas can usually be shown to have metastasized from a primary lesion elsewhere in the body. (REF. 5, p. 930)

205. D. The incidence of diarrhea reported of patients with Zollinger-Ellison syndrome has been variable. One-third to one-half of the patients have been described with this feature. Diarrhea seems to be related to excessive gastric acid production, as it is abolished by total gastrectomy. (REF. 1, pp. 987–988)

206. D. Whipple's disease, formerly believed to be a metabolic lipid disorder, has been more recently recognized as a systemic disease in which clumps and aggregates of large foamy macrophages are found in many organs including the gastrointestinal tract. The cells contain PAS-positive sickle-shaped inclusions. Clinical manifestations include malabsorption syndrome, polyarthritis, and loss of weight. (REF. 1, pp. 848–851)

207. D. The pseudomembranes, which may be focal, punctate, or confluent, are composed of necrotic mucosa admixed with fibrin and polymorphonuclear leukocytes. Other organisms that may cause pseudomembranous colitis include *Shigella, Staphylococcus,* and *Clostridium perfringens.* Prompt administration of vancomycin controls the disease. (REF. 1, p. 327)

208. E. Nodular lymphomas also occur in the gastrointestinal tract. Some lymphomas with a plamacytic component and which produce immunoglobulins (immunoproliferative small cell intestinal lymphomas) are particularly common in the Mediterranean region. (REF. 1, p. 826)

209. E. Fibromuscular hyperplasia of the intestinal arteries, found in elderly individuals, is characterized by intimal thickening and medial proliferation in the terminal parts of the branches of mesenteric arteries just before they enter the bowel. Hypersensitivity to digitalis has been suggested as probable pathogenesis of this lesion. (REF. 1, p. 837)

210. E. Perforation often leads to peritonitis and abscess formation. The iliac veins are most often thrombosed. After 10 or more years of ulcerative colitis, carcinoma tends to develop at multiple sites in the colon. (REF. 1, pp. 860–862)

211. C. Melanosis coli refers to a brownish discoloration of the mucosa of the large intestine. It is due to the accumulation of a melaninlike pigment in mucosal mononuclear cells. The lesion is found in about 10% of autopsies and is associated with chronic constipation and partial obstruction. There is no known significance of this dramatic lesion. (REF. 5, p. 870)

212. A. Venous thrombosis is most often secondary to upper abdominal surgery. Occasionally, slowly developing or incomplete narrowing of the arterial vessels may occur by partial in situ thrombosis or by compression of vessels by adjacent tumor masses, intestinal adhesions, or other mechanical pressures. (REF. 1, p. 831)

213. C. Some have also postulated that the tumor may arise from intercalated duct cells. The neoplasm, though appearing well differentiated histologically, may metastasize; following surgery, 5-year survival rates of 70%–85% have been reported. (REF. 1, p. 793)

214. B. The true mechanism of production of malabsorption state in cases of massive bowel resection and gastroileostomy is failure of absorptive function. In gastroileostomy, the food may bypass the major areas of absorptive surface. (REF. 1, pp. 846–851)

215. D. Warthin's tumor, otherwise known as papillary cyst-adenoma lymphomatosum, is a benign tumor usually found in the major salivary glands. (REF. 1, p. 792)

216. A. Pneumatosis cystoides intestinalis is characterized by gas-filled cysts in the mucosa and wall of the small and large intestine. Predisposing underlying diseases are duodenal ulcer, enterocolitis, and bronchial asthma. The cysts may measure up to 1 cm. The cysts may show a lining of flattened cells or multi-nucleated giant cells. (REF. 2, pp. 1057–1058)

217. C. Actinomycosis, usually caused by *A. israelii*, occurs in three clinical forms: cervicofacial, abdominal, and thoracic. The abdominal involvement consists of inflammation of the appendix and the colon with formation of abscesses and draining sinuses. (REF. 1, pp. 349–350)

218. A. The earliest lesion of typhoid consists of reticuloen-dothelial proliferation of Peyer's patches. Later ulceration of these hypertrophied lymphoid masses leads to the characteristic ovoid ulcers oriented along the long axis of the bowel. (REF. 1, pp. 319–320)

219. B. The damage caused by Shigella organism is usually limited to the colonic mucosa and consists of fibrinosuppurative inflammation with the production of a dirty gray to yellow pseudo-membrane. (REF. 1, p. 322)

220. A. Potassium enteropathy due to local toxicity of potassium chloride tablets occurs in the jejunum and the lesion consists of distinctive focal hemorrhages, congestion, and fibrous thickening of the mucosa. The lesions are sharply segmental and may occur in other parts of the gut. (REF. 2, p. 185)

221. B. The polyps in heredofamilial polyposis are usually small and histologically belong to the pedunculated adenoma type. There is a high incidence of malignant transformation in these polyps. (REF. 1, p. 867)

222. B. Clinically, patients with Whipple's disease show malabsorption syndrome. Pathologically, the mucosa of the small bowel contains numerous macrophages with PAS-positive intracytoplasmic granules. Other organs that may be involved in the disease include the heart, liver, lymph nodes, central nervous system, and skeletal muscle. (REF. 1, p. 848)

223. E. The triad of iron deficiency anemia, dysphagia caused by esophageal webs, and atrophic glossitis is known as Plummer-Vinson syndrome. (REF. 1, pp. 637, 799)

224. A. Autoantibodies to intrinsic factor are also present in the sera of patients with chronic atrophic gastritis. Two types, both IgG, are recognized. (REF. 1, p. 811)

225. A. This refers to one of the microscopic changes in atrophic gastritis consisting of replacement of chief cells by mucin-secreting goblet cells resembling those of the large intestine. (REF. 1, p. 811)

226. B. Several histologic variants of hypertrophic gastritis are described: one with hyperplasia predominantly of surface mucous cells, another with hyperplasia predominantly of glands and an increase in number of parietal cells, and a third type composed of a mixture of both. (REF. 1, p. 812)

227. D. Patients with atrophic gastritis have a predisposition to gastric cancer; approximately 10% will develop this malignancy over the span of decades. (REF. 1, pp. 811–812)

228. D. Granulomatous gastritis is a rare disorder that may occur in sarcoidosis, regional enteritis, or less commonly as an isolated lesion. (REF. 1, p. 813)

229. B. The etiology of tropical sprue is unknown; there are suggestions, however, that the disorder may be derived from intestinal infection. Tropical sprue, though common in the Caribbean, has not been reported in Jamaica. It does not occur in sub-Saharan Africa. (REF. 1, p. 848)

230. D. Macrophages with this description are typically found in Whipple's disease. Additionally the cells contain rod-shaped bacillary bodies. (REF. 1, p. 848)

231. A. Evidence points towards a hereditary basis in some cases of celiac disease. The disease is probably transmitted through a dominant gene with incomplete penetrance. Females are affected more than males. (REF. 1, p. 847)

232. C. The morphologic findings are similar in both tropical and nontropical sprue. By light microscopy there is marked atrophy, distortion, and blunting of the villi of the jejunum. Prominent chronic inflammatory exudate is also observed in the lamina propria. (REF. 1, pp. 847–848)

233. D. These are signs of malabsorption syndrome. As a result of loss of various nutritional components, a motley of deficiencies may ensue. Thus hypoproteinemia, vitamin deficiency, and anemia are usual features of chronic malabsorption. (REF. 1, pp. 846–847)

4 Hepatobiliary System

DIRECTIONS: Each of the questions or incomplete statements below is followed by five suggested answers or completions. Select the **one** that is best in each case.

234. The surface antigen of hepatitis B virus (HB$_s$Ag) is synthesized in hepatocellular
    A. mitochondria
    B. lysosomes
    C. cytoplasm
    D. Golgi apparatus
    E. none of the above

235. The most marked elevation of serum globulin would be encountered in which of the following liver diseases?
    A. Macronodular cirrhosis
    B. Alcoholic cirrhosis
    C. Acute viral hepatitis
    D. Autoimmune type of chronic active hepatitis
    E. Chronic persistent hepatitis

236. Which of the following is least likely to give rise to esophageal varices?
   A. Alcoholic cirrhosis
   B. Postnecrotic cirrhosis
   C. Budd-Chiari syndrome
   D. Pigment cirrhosis
   E. Cardiac cirrhosis

237. Which of the following is NOT true of fatty change?
   A. It is reversible
   B. Fatty change of the liver may be produced by alcoholic injury
   C. In many situations, it represents "unmasking" of the normal fat content of the cells
   D. It may be caused by anoxia alone
   E. Its significance in myocardial stroma is not clear

238. Diffuse liver necrosis most usually occurs with all of the following EXCEPT
   A. infectious mononucleosis
   B. halothane
   C. iproniazid
   D. acute viral hepatitis
   E. eclampsia

239. Acidophilic (Councilman's) bodies are found most frequently in
   A. regular (micronodular) cirrhosis
   B. alcoholic hepatitis
   C. acute viral hepatitis
   D. simple cholestasis
   E. phosphorus liver injury

240. In viral hepatitis, the bridging bands of connective tissue between portal tracts and central veins
   A. are associated with a high frequency of progression to chronic liver disease
   B. indicate better prognosis
   C. are of no significance in prognosis
   D. occur more frequently in children
   E. are often associated with antimitochondrial antibodies

241. The ground-glass appearance of hepatocytic cytoplasm in acute viral hepatitis results from
    A. an increase in smooth endoplasmic reticulum
    B. a decrease in smooth endoplasmic reticulum
    C. an increase in the size of mitochondria
    D. degeneration of intracytoplasmic organelles
    E. none of the above

242. Hepatic injury caused by chlorpromazine is characterized by
    A. nonspecific hepatitis
    B. simple cholestasis
    C. cholestatic hepatitis
    D. granulomatous hepatitis
    E. diffuse steatosis

243. All of the following are true concerning alcoholic liver injury EXCEPT
    A. it occurs in all social classes
    B. characteristic morphologic features are found in the liver
    C. alcoholic liver injury results from associated poor nutrition
    D. alcoholic hepatitis may progress to cirrhosis, but pure fatty liver does not
    E. alcoholic cirrhosis is micronodular (regular)

244. Splenomegaly associated with cirrhosis is
    A. neoplastic
    B. dysplastic
    C. congestive
    D. hamartomatous
    E. inflammatory

245. Which of the following is absent in primary biliary cirrhosis?
    A. Large lymphoid aggregates in the portal tracts
    B. Irregular regeneratory nodules
    C. Prominent plasma cell infiltrate
    D. Bile duct destruction
    E. Cholestasis

246. The most helpful serological test in primary biliary cirrhosis is
  A. antismooth muscle antibodies
  B. antimitochondrial antibodies
  C. HB$_s$Ag
  D. antinuclear antibodies
  E. none of the above

247. All of the following are characterized by indirect bilirubinemia EXCEPT
  A. physiologic jaundice of the newborn
  B. hemolytic disease of the newborn
  C. galactosemia
  D. congenital syphilis
  E. intrahepatic biliary atresia

248. In Reye's syndrome, the liver shows
  A. acute hepatitis
  B. chronic hepatitis
  C. cirrhosis
  D. diffuse steatosis
  E. glycogen storage

249. Hydrops of the gallbladder results from
  A. partial obstruction of the cystic duct
  B. complete obstruction of the cystic duct
  C. partial obstruction of the hepatic duct
  D. complete obstruction of the hepatic duct
  E. obstruction of the common bile duct

250. Which of the following is NOT true of gallbladder carcinoma?
  A. It is more common in whites than blacks
  B. Female–male ratio is 4:1
  C. Gallstones are found in most cases
  D. Indirect bilirubinemia is a common finding
  E. The 5-year survival is low

251. Reduced hepatic cell uptake of bilirubin caused by defects in binding of bilirubin to ligandin Y and ligandin Z is the mechanism of hyperbilirubinemia in

- **A.** Rotor syndrome
- **B.** Dubin-Johnson syndrome
- **C.** Crigler-Najjar syndrome
- **D.** Gilbert's syndrome
- **E.** none of the above

DIRECTIONS: For each of the questions or incomplete statements below, **one** or **more** of the answers or completions given is correct. Select

- **A** if only *1, 2, and 3* are correct
- **B** if only *1 and 3* are correct
- **C** if only *2 and 4* are correct
- **D** if only *4* is correct
- **E** if all are correct

---

252. Which of the following circulatory diseases is (are) located predominantly in the centrilobular zone of the liver?

1. Hemorrhagic necrosis due to hypovolemic shock (shock liver)
2. Budd-Chiari syndrome
3. Chronic passive congestion
4. Zahn's infarct

253. A liver biopsy from "healthy" carriers of hepatitis B virus is most likely to reveal

1. "piecemeal" necrosis
2. intrahepatic cholestasis
3. bile ductular proliferation
4. presence of scattered "ground-glass" hepatocytes

254. Budd-Chiari syndrome has been reported with

1. hepatic cell carcinoma growing into hepatic vein
2. metastatic carcinoma obstructing portal vein
3. adrenal cell carcinoma extending into the hepatic vein
4. polycythemias with portal vein thrombosis

		Directions Summarized		
A	B	C	D	E
1,2,3	1,3	2,4	4	All are
only	only	only	only	correct

255. Which of the following have been implicated in liver cancer in man?
1. Vinyl chloride
2. Carbon tetrachloride
3. Thorotrast
4. *Aspergillus fumigatus*

256. The liver biopsy in alcoholic liver injury may show
1. diffuse steatosis
2. intracytoplasmic hyalin
3. micronodular (regular) cirrhosis
4. sclerosing hyaline necrosis

257. Hepatic veno-occlusive disease is characterized by
1. occlusion of large hepatic vein tributaries
2. occlusion of centrilobular and sublobular hepatic veins
3. prevalence among Eskimos
4. association with ingestion of natural hepatotoxins

258. Which of the following (is) are true concerning neonatal (giant cell) hepatitis?
1. Hepatitis-associated antigen is invariably positive
2. It may occur in biliary atresia
3. It often progresses to infantile cirrhosis
4. It may be encountered in cytomegalic inclusion disease

259. Fatty liver of pregnancy
1. usually occurs in the second trimester of pregnancy
2. runs a benign course
3. incidence is about 1 per 500 pregnancies
4. may follow intravenous tetracycline therapy

260. Macronodular gross morphology is typical of cirrhosis
1. following chronic active hepatitis
2. associated with hemochromatosis (pigment cirrhosis)
3. associated with Wilson's disease
4. of alcoholic etiology

261. Significantly elevated levels of which of the following occurs in primary hepatocellular carcinoma?
1. Carcinoembryonic antigen
2. Ceruloplasmin
3. Alpha-1 antitrypsin
4. Alpha fetoprotein

DIRECTIONS: The group of questions below consists of five lettered headings followed by a list of numbered words, phrases, or statements. For **each** numbered word, phrase, or statement, select the **one** lettered heading that is most closely associated with it. Each lettered heading may be selected once, more than once, or not at all.

Questions 262–265:
A. HB_sAg (surface antigen of hepatitis B)
B. HB_eAg (e antigen)
C. HB_cAg (core antigen)
D. antiHBe (antibody to e antigen)
E. antiHB$_s$ (antibody to surface antigen)

262. Earliest marker of acute infection with hepatitis B virus

263. Rising titers during the "window period"

264. Confers life-long immunity

265. Physicochemical similarity to IgG_4 immunoglobulin

Questions 266–272:
A. Cholestasis and necrosis
B. Simple cholestasis
C. Massive necrosis
D. Steatosis
E. Micronodular (regular) cirrhosis

266. Methotrexate

267. Phenothiazines

268. Azathioprine

269. Oral contraceptives

270. Halothane

271. Tetracycline

272. Testosterone

DIRECTIONS: The set of lettered headings below is followed by a list of numbered words or phrases. For each numbered word or phrase select

A   if the item is associated with (A) *only*
B   if the item is associated with (B) *only*
C   if the item is associated with *both* (A) *and* (B)
D   if the item is associated with *neither* (A) *nor* (B)

Questions 273–279:
   A.   Hepatitis A virus
   B.   Hepatitis B virus
   C.   Both
   D.   Neither

273. Enterovirus

274. Dane particle

275. Chronic aggressive hepatitis

276. Most cases of posttransfusion hepatitis

277. Acute lesion showing acidophilic (Councilman's) bodies and ballooning degeneration

278. Subacute hepatic necrosis with bridging

279. e antigen

Answers and Comments

234. C. The complete hepatitis B virion, also called the Dane particle, measures 42 nm and is composed of an inner core measuring 27 nm, surrounded by an outer coat. The core is synthesized in the hepatocellular nucleus. (REF. 1, p. 901)

235. D. The elevation of the globulin fraction is due to an increase in the gamma-globulin fraction. In chronic active hepatitis, IgG is significantly elevated. (REF. 3, pp. 232–233)

236. E. Esophageal varices are caused by portal hypertension, in which portal blood flow is diverted through the coronary veins of the stomach into esophageal submucosal veins and from there to the azygous system of veins. (REF. 1, pp. 802–803)

237. C. There has to be a substantial absolute increase in the intracellular fat content before fat vacuoles are visible under light microscopy. (REF. 1, pp. 18–21)

238. E. Eclampsia produces predominantly periportal necrosis. (REF. 1, p. 1156)

239. C. Acidophilic bodies are hepatocytes that have undergone a peculiar coagulative change and appear as round, anuclear, eosinophilic inclusion. Sometimes they are called Councilman's bodies. (REF. 1, p. 906)

240. A. In viral hepatitis, when such bridging occurs, the lesion is referred to as subacute hepatic necrosis. It is associated with a high frequency of progression to cirrhosis. (REF. 1, p. 906)

241. A. Ground-glass appearance of hepatocytes in acute viral hepatitis may also be found after exposure to many drugs and chemicals, including pesticides. (REF. 1, p. 905)

242. C. The effect of chlorpromazine on the liver is not predictable and the incidence of cholestatic hepatitis secondary to chlorpromazine injury is about 1%. Clinically, manifestations of hypersensitivity may accompany liver derangements. (REF. 1, p. 914)

243. C. It has been shown in both humans and baboons that alcohol is toxic to the liver. Alcohol affects the oxidative capacity of hepatocytes and causes swelling of the mitochondria and endoplasmic reticulum. (REF. 1, pp. 917–920)

244. C. Grossly, the spleen in liver cirrhosis is firm, dark red, and may weigh between 300 g and 1000 g. There is a little correlation between the size of the spleen and increased pressure in the portal system. (REF. 1, p. 917)

245. B. Biliary cirrhosis results in a very finely and diffusely nodular liver. In secondary biliary cirrhosis the liver is also intensely green. In neither of the two types are irregular nodules found. (REF. 1, p. 929)

246. B. Antismooth muscle antibodies may be positive in primary biliary cirrhosis but are of greatest use in chronic active hepatitis. (REF. 1, p. 930)

247. E. Intrahepatic biliary atresia causes obstruction and direct hyperbilirubincmia. (REF. 1, p. 895)

248. D. The etiology of Reye's syndrome is not known. It usually begins as an upper respiratory tract infection, followed by vomiting, delirium, and coma. The liver shows fatty vacuoles of the fine foamy type. (REF. 1, pp. 941–942)

249. B. Grossly, the gallbladder is tense and enlarged and has a translucent appearance; the lumen contains a clear, watery mucous secretion; microscopically, there may be mucosal atrophy. (REF. 1, p. 951)

250. D. Obstruction of the bile ducts would cause direct bilirubinemia, which is not true of gallbladder carcinoma. (REF. 1, p. 951)

251. D. In some cases of Gilbert's syndrome, glucuronyl transferase is also reduced. The disease is harmless, producing no symptoms or occasional mild jaundice. Liver biopsy is normal. (REF. 2, p. 1156)

252. E. Zahn's infarct is a localized area of redness due to marked sinusoidal congestion. Hepatocellular atrophy rather than necrosis is present. The lesion may be caused by occlusion of an intrahepatic branch of the portal vein. (REF. 1, pp. 896–899)

253. D. "Ground-glass" hepatocytes are seen as enlarged finely granular eosinophilic cytoplasm. The presence of HB_sAg in these cells can be demonstrated by orcein or aldehyde fuchsin stains or by immunofluorescence or immunoperoxidase techniques. (REF. 1, pp. 904–905)

254. B. Budd-Chiari syndrome is caused by occlusive lesions of the hepatic veins. Such occlusion has been reported with a large number of primary and metastatic carcinomas of the liver and other tumors of the retroperitoneum, including those arising from adrenal glands. Thrombosis and obstruction of the portal vein do not cause the enlargement of the liver and the impairment of hepatic function produced by severe congestion as is seen in Budd-Chiari syndrome. (REF. 2, pp. 1176–1177)

255. B. Thorotrast, which was used in diagnostic radiology, has been associated with hemangioendothelioma and hepatocarcinoma. Vinyl chloride has more recently been implicated in hepatic angiosarcoma. (REF. 2, pp. 182–185)

256. E. In addition to the listed features, intracytoplasmic hyalin may be present in alcohol-induced liver injury. (REF. 1, pp. 918–920)

257. C. The ingestion of "bush tea" containing senecio alkaloids is known to precipitate hepatic veno-occlusive disease. The disease is characterized by hepatomegaly, ascites, and sudden onset of abdominal enlargement. It occurs most commonly between the ages of 18 months and 3 years. (REF. 2, p. 1177)

258. C. Giant cell transformation of the liver may occur in hemolytic disease of the newborn, cytomegalic inclusion disease, and congenital syphilis. However, in the majority of cases, no specific etiology can be identified. (REF. 1, p. 940)

259. D. Fatty liver of pregnancy is a rare, highly fatal disease that occurs in the third trimester. Most cases are of idiopathic origin but may follow intravenous tetracycline therapy. (REF. 2, p. 1169)

260. B. In macronodular (irregular) cirrhosis, regeneratory nodules are irregular and large, reaching up to 3–5 cm in diameter. The fibrous septa are broad. The term "post-necrotic" cirrhosis is also frequently used to describe this entity. (REF. 1, p. 923)

261. D. Significantly elevated serum levels of alpha fetoprotein are observed in more than two-thirds of patients with hepatocellular carcinoma. High levels of this protein may also be observed in patients with yolk sac tumors and massive hepatic necrosis. (REF. 1, p. 938)

262. A. Titers of HB$_s$Ag usually disappear with resolution of acute hepatitis; persistence of antigen suggests progression to chronic liver disease. (REF. 1, p. 902)

263. D. The "window" refers to the period between the disappearance of HB$_s$Ag and the appearance of anti-HB$_s$. In addition to the rising titers of anti-HB$_e$, anti-HB$_c$ may also be detected during this period. (REF. 1, p. 902)

264. E. Anti-HB$_s$ is detectable in the serum week to months ("window") after the disappearance of HB$_s$Ag. (REF. 1, pp. 901–902)

265. B. The e antigen is immunologically distinct from both HB$_s$Ag and HB$_c$Ag. The e antigen indicates infectivity and is usually detectable in the serum when HB$_s$Ag is also present. (REF. 1, pp. 901–902)

266. E. When used for many years, especially in the treatment of psoriasis, methotrexate causes regular cirrhosis with little steatosis but conspicuous enlargement of hepatocytes and their nuclei. (REF. 1, p. 914)

267. A. Phenothiazines cause cholestatic hepatitis. This injury is nonpredictable. Other drugs that cause cholestatic hepatitis are sulfonylurea, azathioprine, and organic arsenicals. (REF. 1, p. 914)

268. A. See explanatory answer 267. (REF. 1, p. 914)

269. B. Cholestasis induced by drugs is mainly centrilobular in location. Other drugs causing the same reaction are methyltestosterone and some other anabolic steroids. (REF. 1, p. 914)

270. C. Halothane causes a drug hepatitis almost indistinguishable from acute viral hepatitis. Other drugs prone to produce similar lesions include cinchophen iproniazid and monoamine oxidase inhibitors. (REF. 1, p. 914)

271. D. This reaction in the liver is predictable. (REF. 1, p. 914)

272. B. Testosterone causes simple cholestasis. (REF. 1, p. 914)

273. A. Hepatitis A virus, first isolated in 1973, is most probably an entero- or picornavirus. The virion is a homogenous particle with cubic symmetry. (REF. 1, p. 900)

274. B. The complete infectious virion of hepatitis B — called the Dane particle—consists of an inner core 27 nm in diameter composed of circular DNA 70% of which is double-stranded and the remainder single-stranded. Also found within the core particle are hepatitis B core antigen and DNA-dependent polymerase. (REF. 1, p. 901)

275. B. Also called chronic active hepatitis, this liver disorder, characterized by lymphocytic infiltration of portal tracts with periportal necrosis and inflammation (piecemeal necrosis), may also be caused by drugs such as methyldopa and isoniazid, by Wilson's disease, and alpha-1-antitrypsin deficiency. (REF. 1, p. 907)

276. D. About 90% of posttransfusion hepatitis is caused by the so-called non-A non-B virus. Although the virus has not been isolated, the disease has been transmitted by injection of serum into chimpanzees. (REF. 1, p. 903)

277. C. Acute hepatitis caused by A, B, or non-A non-B virus shows similar morphologic features. There is a focal or spotty cytolytic lobular necrosis, reticuloendothelial and lymphocytic response, and evidence of regeneration. (REF. 1, p. 906)

278. B. This consists of septa of confluent necrosis linking central veins to each other and to adjacent portal tracts. The disease may be fatal; many patients who survive may develop chronic active hepatitis and cirrhosis. (REF. 1, p. 906)

279. B. HB$_e$Ag, a protein that resembles an immunoglobulin, may be detected in acute serum as well as in chronic carriers. The antigen seems to be associated with a high degree of infectivity and in chronic carriers, a likelihood of progressive liver disease. (REF. 1, p. 902)

5 Respiratory System

DIRECTIONS: Each of the questions or incomplete statements below is followed by five suggested answers or completions. Select the **one** that is best in each case.

280. All of the following statements concerning pulmonary tuberculosis are true EXCEPT
    A. black people and American Indians are more susceptible than Caucasians
    B. "hard" tuberculous granulomas may be difficult to distinguish from granulomas of sarcoidosis
    C. the Ghon complex is composed of a primary pulmonary lesion associated with regional lymph node involvement
    D. the initial lesion of primary tuberculosis is located at the apex of the lung
    E. the erosion of pulmonary artery by a tuberculous focus causes predominantly miliary pulmonary spread

281. The Reid index is useful in the microscopic diagnosis of
    A. acute bronchitis
    B. bronchiectasis
    C. chronic bronchitis
    D. pulmonary emphysema
    E. bronchial asthma

282. All of the following may be found in a patient with intrinsic bronchial asthma EXCEPT
   A. Curschmann's spirals in the sputum
   B. Charcot-Leyden crystals in the sputum
   C. eosinophils in the sputum
   D. hypertrophy of bronchial smooth muscle
   E. increased IgE levels

283. Which of the following morphological features is usually NOT seen in viral pneumonitis?
   A. Mononuclear and histiocytic infiltrate in the alveolar spaces
   B. Focal necrosis of alveolar walls
   C. Hyaline membrane formation
   D. Fibrin thrombi in capillaries
   E. Thickened septal walls

284. A 40-year-old engineer presents with enlarged hilar lymph nodes, hepatosplenomegaly, hypercalcemia, and interstitial lung disease. The most probable diagnosis is
   A. hyperparathyroidism
   B. leukemia
   C. histoplasmosis
   D. sarcoidosis
   E. tuberculosis

285. Which of the following characteristically shows macroscopic nodularity?
   A. Anthracosis
   B. Silicosis
   C. Berylliosis
   D. Silo filler's disease
   E. Asbestosis

286. Which is the most common hormone or hormonelike substance produced by pulmonary carcinoma?
   A. ACTH or ACTH-like substance
   B. ADH
   C. Gonadotropin
   D. Parathormone
   E. Melanocyte-stimulating hormone

287. Which tumor of the lung has the poorest prognosis?
     A. Small cell (oat cell) carcinoma
     B. Squamous cell carcinoma
     C. Malignant lymphoma
     D. Adenocarcinoma
     E. Bronchiolo-alveolar carcinoma

288. A pulmonary carcinoma arising in an area of scarring would most probably be
     A. squamous cell carcinoma
     B. oat cell carcinoma
     C. giant cell carcinoma
     D. cylindroma
     E. adenocarcinoma

289. Interstitial pulmonary fibrosis may be caused by all of the following EXCEPT
     A. sarcoidosis
     B. progressive systemic sclerosis (scleroderma)
     C. berylliosis
     D. radiation
     E. bronchial asthma

290. Which one of the following should be strongly suspected in bronchiectasis that is associated with parasinusitis?
     A. Cystic fibrosis
     B. Kartagener's syndrome
     C. Agammaglobulinemia
     D. Status post-pertussis infection
     E. Status post-recurrent episodes of pneumonitis

291. Most of the cells that fill the alveoli in desquamative interstitial pneumonitis are
     A. plasma cells
     B. lymphocytes
     C. macrophages
     D. neutrophils
     E. fibroblasts

DIRECTIONS: For each of the questions or incomplete statements below, **one** or **more** of the answers or completions given is correct. Select

    A if only *1, 2, and 3* are correct
    B if only *1 and 3* are correct
    C if only *2 and 4* are correct
    D if only *4* is correct
    E if all are correct

292. Polyps of the larynx
    1. are synonymous with papillomas of the larynx
    2. may also be called "singer's nodes"
    3. have a propensity for malignant change
    4. occur most often on the true vocal cords

293. Pulmonary hypertension may be caused by
    1. mitral stenosis
    2. Eisenmenger's complex
    3. left ventricular failure
    4. kyphoscoliosis

294. "Ferruginous bodies" are usually found in
    1. silicosis
    2. siderosilicosis
    3. pulmonary hemosiderosis
    4. asbestosis

295. Honeycomb lung may be found in
    1. sarcoidosis
    2. carcinomatous lymphangitis
    3. Hamman-Rich syndrome
    4. organizing bronchopneumonia

296. Which of the following drugs may cause interstitial pulmonary fibrosis?
 1. Busulfan
 2. Methotrexate
 3. Hexamethonium
 4. Prednisolone

297. Which of the following may be found in infection with *Pneumocystis carinii* pneumonia?
 1. Interstitial pneumonia with plasma cell infiltrate
 2. Granulomatous inflammation of the lung
 3. Disseminated disease in spleen, liver, and lymph nodes
 4. Pulmonary abscess

298. The most significant pathologic alteration(s) in chronic bronchitis is (are)
 1. hyperplasia of bronchial mucosal glands
 2. smooth muscle hypertrophy
 3. goblet cell hyperplasia
 4. eosinophilic infiltration of the bronchial wall

299. Wegener's granulomatosis is characterized by
 1. necrotizing granuloma in the upper respiratory tract and lung
 2. vasculitis of small vessels
 3. glomerulonephritis
 4. pulmonary hemorrhage with epitheloid granulomas

300. Severe pulmonary hypertension is indicated by
 1. intimal thickening of muscular arteries
 2. plexiform lesions occurring in muscular arteries
 3. medial hypertrophy of muscular arteries
 4. necrotizing arteritis

301. "Brown induration" of the lung may be present in
 1. congestive heart failure
 2. Goodpasture's syndrome
 3. idiopathic hemosiderosis
 4. mechanical obstruction of pulmonary veins

		Directions Summarized		
A	B	C	D	E
1,2,3	1,3	2,4	4	All are
only	only	only	only	correct

302. Pulmonary tuberculosis may be caused by
1. *Mycobacterium tuberculosis*
2. *Mycobacterium scrofulaceum*
3. *Mycobacterium kansasii*
4. *Mycobacterium ulcerans*

DIRECTIONS: Each group of questions below consists of five lettered headings followed by a list of numbered words, phrases, or statements. For **each** numbered word, phrase, or statement, select the **one** lettered heading that is most closely associated with it. Each lettered heading may be selected once, more than once, or not at all.

Questions 303–309:
A. Asbestosis
B. Berylliosis
C. Bagassosis
D. Anthracosis
E. Silicosis

303. Complicated by tuberculosis

304. Dense fibrocollagenous tissue arranged in concentric bands containing crystals visualized by polarized light

305. Fibers measuring $0.5 \, \mu \times 50 \, \mu$

306. Mesothelioma

307. Sandblasting

308. Hypersensitivity pneumonitis

309. Sarcoidlike granulomas with Schaumann bodies

Questions 310–316:
- A. Pulmonary adenocarcinoma
- B. Squamous cell carcinoma of the lung
- C. Small cell anaplastic "oat cell" carcinoma
- D. Bronchiolar (alveolar cell) carcinoma
- E. Mesothelioma

310. Tumor cells contain acid mucopolysaccharides which can be stained with Alcian blue

311. Neurosecretory granules demonstrable by electron microscopy

312. Most closely associated with smoking history

313. Most likely to produce ACTH and/or ADH

314. Most closely related to the bronchial carcinoid

315. Histologically resembles the infectious disease of South African sheep known as jagziekte

316. Most commonly associated with ferruginous bodies

DIRECTIONS: Each set of lettered headings below is followed by a list of numbered words or phrases. For each numbered word or phrase select
- A if the item is associated with (A) *only*
- B if the item is associated with (B) *only*
- C if the item is associated with *both* (A) *and* (B)
- D if the item is associated with *neither* (A) *nor* (B)

Questions 317–321:
- A. Centriacinar (centrilobular) emphysema
- B. Panacinar (panlobular) emphysema
- C. Both
- D. Neither

317. More commonly associated with alpha-1-antitrypsin deficiency

318. Emphysematous bullae

319. Honeycomb lung

320. Selective and predominant destruction of respiratory bronchioles

321. Senile emphysema

Answers and Comments

280. D. The Ghon focus, which represents the initial pulmonary tuberculous infection, is a subpleural lesion which is located either just above or just below the interlobar fissure between the upper and the lower lobes. The initial lesion of secondary or reinfection tuberculosis, on the other hand, is found in the apical regions of the lung. (REF. 1, p. 342)

281. C. The Reid index is the ratio of the thickness of the bronchial mucous glands to the thickness of the wall (the gland/wall ratio). This is normally 0.14 to 0.36 but may be as high as 0.79 in chronic bronchitis. (REF. 1, p. 726)

282. E. Elevated IgE levels are characteristically present in extrinsic bronchial asthma. After antigenic stimulus, IgE is produced and fixes to human basophils and tissue mast cells. A challenge dose of antigen causes release of vasoactive agents from the sensitized mast cells and leads to the activation of chemical mediators. Together these mediators cause the contraction of smooth muscle, especially that of the bronchi in the asthmatic. (REF. 1, p. 727)

283. A. The seat of the disease process in viral pneumonitis is the alveolar wall. The inflammatory infiltrate, predominantly mononuclear, is found in the alveolar walls and not in the alveoli themselves. (REF. 1, p. 737)

284. D. Sarcoidosis is a disease of unknown etiology characterized pathologically by non-necrotizing epitheloid granulomata, which may occur in any organ or tissue. About 75% of cases are asymptomatic. The most frequently involved sites are the lymph nodes, spleen, liver, lungs, and bone. (REF. 1, pp. 390–392)

285. B. Macroscopic nodularity gives silicosis a unique appearance among the pneumoconioses. The nodules are fibrous and slowly increase in size until they can be recognized on roentgenographic examination. Microscopically, the nodules are composed of collagenized and densely hyalinized tissue arranged in concentric bands; inflammatory reaction is absent. Silica crystals within the nodules may be visualized with polarized light. (REF. 1, p. 436)

286. A. Nearly all the endocrine syndromes are associated with oat cell carcinoma but the most common is Cushing's syndrome, which is of sudden onset and may be fulminant. The same syndrome may be associated with bronchial carcinoid. (REF. 1, p. 754)

287. A. Small cell carcinoma of the lung is characterized by diffuse sheets of closely packed cells about the size of lymphocytes. Many are round and ovoid, but fusiform forms are not uncommon. Recently the endocrine potential of some of these tumors and a close resemblance to carcinoid have been recognized. (REF. 1, p. 754)

288. E. Chronic inflammation and fibrosis in the lung are associated with two types of tumors: the tumorlet and adenocarcinoma. The tumorlet, considered by some as minute carcinoma, ranges from microscopic size to about 3 mm in diameter. It must be distinguished from pulmonary peripheral carcinoid and pulmonary chemodectoma. About two-thirds of lung scar adenocarcinomas are less than 3 cm in diameter. Most are subpleural and appear as puckered scars and their incidence has not been determined. (REF. 1, p. 751)

289. E. The cardinal anatomic changes in bronchial asthma are found in the bronchioles and bronchi, which contain tenacious mucous plugs. Microscopically, such plugs contain Curschmann's spirals. Charcot-Leyden crystals, and eosinophils. The bronchial mucosa is edematous and contains inflammatory cells, including many eosinophils. (REF. 1, pp. 727, 747)

290. B. Kartagener's syndrome includes bronchiectasis, parasinusitis, and situs inversus. (REF. 1, p. 729)

291. C. By electron microscopy, approximately 90% of desquamated cells are histiocytes (macrophages), many containing intracytoplasmic lipid and PAS-positive granules. They are most probably derived from alveolar pneumocytes type II. (REF. 1, p. 747)

292. C. Laryngeal polyps are inflammatory overgrowths that occur most frequently on the true vocal cords. Microscopically, the polyps are composed of a core of vascularized connective tissue within which inflammatory cells are scattered and which is covered with stratified squamous epithelium. (REF. 1, p. 761)

293. E. Other causes of pulmonary hypertension are patent ductus arteriosus, atrial or ventricular septal defect, multiple and recurrent pulmonary emboli, emphysema, many pneumoconioses, and pulmonary fibrosis. (REF. 2, pp. 866–870)

294. D. Controversy exists as to whether ferruginous bodies should be regarded as asbestos bodies. In many cases the underlying core of these bodies has been shown to lack chrysotile, one of the forms in which asbestos is found in human body. (REF. 1, p. 438)

295. B. The essential change in honeycomb lung is obliteration, by fibrosis or granuloma, of some of the bronchioles and their subdivisions. Neighboring unaffected bronchioles undergo compensatory dilation, forming cysts next to consolidated or fibrotic areas that may cause interstitial pulmonary fibrosis. (REF. 1, p. 743)

296. B. Other drugs that may cause interstitial pulmonary fibrosis are nitrofurantoin, methysergide, oxygen, and bleomycin. (REF. 1, pp. 894–895)

297. A. Disseminated pneumocystosis may occur in the lymph nodes, liver, spleen, and bone marrow. (REF. 1, pp. 365–366)

298. B. Submucosal glands are hyperplastic and can be expressed as an increased Reid index. The changes in the glands are also responsible for the production of sputum, a hallmark of chronic bronchitis. (REF. 1, p. 726)

299. A. Clinically, Wegener's granulomatosis manifests as intractable rhinitis and sinusitis, nodular pulmonary lesions with cough and hemoptysis, and terminal uremia. The pathologic findings in the kidney include focal necrotizing glomerulitis, fibrinous necrosis, crescent formation, and vasculitis. (REF. 1, pp. 523–524)

300. C. Plexiform and angiomatoid lesions of muscular arteries with or without necrotizing arteritis may occur in primary pulmonary hypertension. They may also be found, however, in pulmonary hypertension secondary to congenital cardiac disease with shunt and in pulmonary schistosomiasis. (REF. 2, p. 867)

301. E. Regarding brown induration, in all options listed, the lungs are rubbery and brown. The color change is due to the presence of hemosiderin-laden macrophages within the alveolar spaces, which may lead to interstitial fibrosis. (REF. 1, p. 711)

302. B. *Mycobacterium ulcerans* is the cause of Buruli ulcers, a superficial ulceration of the skin with associated fat necrosis. Systemic manifestations are not known. *Mycobacterium scrofulaceum* causes predominantly acute and subacute lymphadenitis. (REF. 1, p. 346)

303. E. Silicosis with tuberculosis is a variant of silicosis occurring in up to two-thirds of patients with silicosis as reported in some studies; in others, an incidence of about 10% is reported. There appears to be a synergism between silica and the tubercule bacilli. (REF. 1, p. 436)

304. E. Grossly, such lungs show diffuse nodularity, a characteristic feature of this pneumoconiosis. (REF. 1, p. 436)

305. A. The largest irritant particles are probably found in this disease. Subsequently, diffuse pulmonary fibrosis results. Complications or long-term sequelae include bronchogenic carcinoma and mesothelioma. (REF. 1, p. 460)

306. A. A survey of 52 cases of pleural mesothelioma revealed a history of exposure to asbestos in 80% of the patients. A firm diagnosis can be made only if a thorough search fails to reveal a primary tumor elsewhere in the body. (REF. 1, pp. 760–761)

307. E. Other workers who face the hazard of silicosis are stonemasons, boiler scalers, and those preparing clay for the manufacture of pottery. (REF. 1, p. 436)

308. C. The cause of this disease is a thermophilic actinomycetes. The disease may progress to interstitial fibrosis. (REF. 2, p. 878)

309. B. Acute berylliosis is an acute chemical pneumonitis. Granulomas are not formed during this phase of the illness. The granulomas of chronic berylliosis are found predominantly in the pulmonary system but may be found in the liver, spleen, lymph nodes, and skin. (REF. 1, pp. 440 – 442)

310. E. Microscopically, the mesothelioma is composed of two types of tissues (biphasic pattern): mesenchymal stromal cells and/or epithelial-like cells. The overall histologic morphology depends on the proportion of these two types of cells ranging from a picture resembling spindle cell sarcoma to one suggestive of a pure carcinoma. (REF. 1, p. 760)

311. C. The precise histogenesis of "oat cell" carcinoma of the lung remains unsettled but the cells are most probably derived from Kulchitsky cells, known to be present in neonatal human bronchial epithelium. (REF. 1, p. 752)

312. B. Squamous cell carcinoma is also most commonly found in men. The tumor is usually located in the central part of the lung—generally the first, second, and third order bronchi. (REF. 1, p. 753)

313. C. Inappropriate hormonal secretion has been associated with all histological types of lung cancer. Hormones elaborated include parathormone inducing hypercalcemia, calcitonin causing hypocalcemia, and gonadotropins causing gynecomastia. (REF. 1, p. 754)

314. C. Bronchial carcinoids arise from Kulchitsky cells of the bronchial epithelium; the tumor cells on electron microscopy contain membrane-bound neurosecretory granules. They are slow-growing tumors but may metastasize. (REF. 1, p. 755)

315. D. Histologically, the alveolar spaces and the terminal bronchioles are lined by tall columnar to cuboidal tumor cells that often contain abundant mucus. The native septal architecture of the lung is usually preserved. The tumor may occur as single nodules located in the periphery of the lung but more often as multiple nodules which are sometimes confluent. Diffuse involvement of large areas of a lung lobe or an entire lung is not unusual. (REF. 1, p. 755)

316. E. There is an etiologic relationship between heavy asbestos exposure and mesothelioma. Ferruginous bodies are asbestos fibers coated with acid mucopolysaccharide or protein on which iron granules, most probably ferritin, are deposited. (REF. 1, p. 760)

317. B. Patients with homozygous (PiZZ) alpha-1-antitrypsin deficiency have extremely low serum levels of the enzyme and greatly enhanced susceptibility to pulmonary emphysema. In these patients, emphysema is characteristically found in a younger age group and the disease tends to be severe and localized in the lower lobes. (REF. 1, pp. 721–722)

318. C. Bullae are emphysematous spaces greater than 1 cm in diameter. They are usually subpleural and represent localized accentuation of any of the destructive emphysematous processes. (REF. 1, p. 723)

319. D. The end stage of diffuse interstial diseases shows severe interstitial fibrosis, gross destruction of the lung, and bronchiolar dilatation, a constellation of changes called "honeycomb" lung. It should be noted that pulmonary emphysema does not show fibrosis and inflammatory changes. (REF. 1, p. 748)

320. A. This accurately defines centriacinar emphysema. Panacinar emphysema, on the other hand, is characterized by uniform enlargement and destruction of the entire acinus. (REF. 1, p. 718)

321. D. Senile emphysema is a compensatory hyperinflation of the lung in which there is destruction of lung parenchyma. The alveolar ducts and respiratory bronchioles enlarge with age while the alveoli become smaller and shallower. (REF. 1, p. 724)

6 Genitourinary and Pediatric Pathology

322. In the presence of a barely palpable testicular tumor, gynecomastia, and large pulmonary metastasis in a 30-year-old man, the most likely diagnosis is
    A. seminoma
    B. adult teratoma
    C. teratocarcinoma
    D. choriocarcinoma
    E. Leydig cell tumor

323. When the nephrotic syndrome occurs in a diabetic, the renal biopsy typically shows
    A. nodular glomerulosclerosis
    B. diffuse glomerulosclerosis
    C. necrotizing papillitis
    D. acute pyelonephritis
    E. chronic pyelonephritis

324. All of the following are true concerning renal artery stenosis EXCEPT
  - **A.** atheromatous plaque obstructing the origin of the renal artery is the most common cause
  - **B.** fibromuscular dysplasia causing renal artery stenosis may affect the intima, media, or adventitia
  - **C.** arterioles in the affected kidney typically show hypertensive changes
  - **D.** the juxtaglomerular apparatus undergoes hyperplasia
  - **E.** the kidney is usually small due to ischemic atrophy

325. Proliferative glomerular changes are observed in all of the following EXCEPT
  - **A.** Fanconi syndrome
  - **B.** bacterial endocarditis
  - **C.** Henoch-Schönlein purpura
  - **D.** lupus erythematosus
  - **E.** Wegener's granulomatosis

326. The pathology of the kidney in multiple myeloma principally involves
  - **A.** the glomeruli
  - **B.** the interstitium
  - **C.** rcnal arteries
  - **D.** renal veins
  - **E.** the tubules

327. Dense deposit disease refers to
  - **A.** IgG-IgA Berger's nephropathy
  - **B.** renal amyloidosis
  - **C.** a subgroup of membranoproliferative glomerulonephritis
  - **D.** a subgroup of postinfectious proliferative glomerulonephritis
  - **E.** a subgroup of rapidly progressive glomerulonephritis

328. Renal involvement in systemic lupus erythematosus does NOT manifest as
    A. plugging of renal tubules with proteinaceous cast evoking a giant cell reaction
    B. proliferative glomerulonephritis
    C. focal glomerulonephritis
    D. membranous nephropathy
    E. crescentic glomerulonephritis

329. Which of the following is the classic morphological manifestation of membranous nephropathy?
    A. Subepithelial deposits of electron-dense material and "spikes"
    B. Crescent formation
    C. Adhesion formation between glomerula tuft and Bowman's capsule
    D. Nodular sclerosis of glomerular tuft
    E. Inflammatory exudate and necrosis of capillary loops

330. Light microscopy of renal tubular epithelium may permit the diagnosis of which of the following?
    A. Hyponatremia
    B. Hypokalemia
    C. Hypernatremia
    D. Hyperkalemia
    E. Azotemia

331. Which of the following is NOT characteristic of Goodpasture's syndrome?
    A. Pulmonary hemorrhages
    B. Clinical evidence of renal disease
    C. Rapidly progressive disorder
    D. Occurrence in young adults, especially in men
    E. Deposition of subepithelial humps in glomeruli

332. Which of the following rules out the diagnosis of Stein-Leventhal syndrome?
    A. Infertility
    B. Hirsutism
    C. Oligomenorrhea
    D. Involuted corpus luteum
    E. Occurrence in late teens and early twenties

333. The characteristic feature of malakoplakia is the presence of von Hansemann cells and
    A. calcium phosphate precipitates on damaged mucosal surface
    B. Michaelis-Gutmann bodies
    C. von Brunn's nests
    D. calcified eggs of *Schistosoma haematobium*
    E. Schaumann bodies

334. Which of the following histologic features is NOT seen in salpingitis isthmica nodosa?
    A. Bundles of smooth muscle separate glandular channels and spaces
    B. Benign tubal epithelium lines the channels
    C. Plasmacytic, lymphocytic, and histiocytic infiltrate is abundant and extensively involves the tubal lumen and wall
    D. Glandular channels communicate with the tubal lumen
    E. Inflammatory changes are inconspicuous or absent

335. A testicular lesion in which Reinke crytalloids are found is most likely to be a(n)
    A. Sertoli cell tumor
    B. adenomatoid tumor
    C. seminoma
    D. Leydig cell tumor
    E. endodermal sinus tumor

336. Alpha-fetoprotein would be most frequently demonstrable in which tumor of the testis?
    A. Choriocarcinoma
    B. Seminoma
    C. Endodermal sinus tumor
    D. Granulosa cell tumor
    E. Immature teratoma

337. The kidney biopsy in IgA nephropathy most commonly shows
    A. diffuse proliferative glomerulonephritis
    B. focal glomerulonephritis
    C. crescentic glomerulonephritis
    D. mesangioproliferative glomerulonephritis
    E. no changes by light microscopy

338. Which of the following statements is incorrect regarding the nature of glomerular crescents?
    A. They arise from the proliferation of visceral epithelial cells
    B. The presence of crescents signifies severe progressive renal disease
    C. There are focal disruptions in glomerular basement membrane
    D. Macrophages form an integral part of crescents
    E. Crescent formation is typically found in Goodpasture's syndrome

339. Factors predisposing to endometrial adenocarcinoma include the following EXCEPT
    A. nulliparity
    B. diabetes mellitus
    C. hypertension
    D. oral contraceptives
    E. prolonged treatment with high doses of estrogen

340. Which of the following cyclical endometrial changes suggest combined estrogen and progesterone effect?
    A. Tubular endometrial glands
    B. Compact endometrial stroma
    C. Abundant gland mitoses
    D. Basal vacuolation
    E. Nonalignment of glandular nuclei

341. Pseudomyxoma peritonei may be expected to arise from which ovarian neoplasm?
    A. Mucinous cystadenocarcinoma
    B. Endometrial adenocarcinoma
    C. Serous cystadenocarcinoma
    D. Clear cell adenocarcinoma
    E. Undifferentiated carcinoma

342. All of the following statements concerning malignant germ cell tumors of the testis are true EXCEPT
    A. tests for chorionic gonadotropin should be performed in every patient suspected of having a testicular tumor
    B. the blood and urine of some patients may contain large amounts of follicle-stimulating hormone
    C. pure choriocarcinomas are the most malignant
    D. prognosis is worse when choriocarcinoma is associated with other germ cell tumors
    E. seminomas are the most radiosensitive

DIRECTIONS: For each of the questions or incomplete statements below, **one** or **more** of the answers or completions given is correct. Select

   A if only *1, 2, and 3* are correct
   B if only *1 and 3* are correct
   C if only *2 and 4* are correct
   D if only *4* is correct
   E if all are correct

---

343. Classic carcinoid syndrome is associated with
    1. carcinoid of the appendix
    2. carcinoid of the ileum with hepatic metastasis
    3. carcinoid of the sigmoid with regional lymph node metastasis
    4. carcinoid of the ovary

344. Which of the following ovarian tumor(s) has (have) been associated with endometrial adenocarcinoma?
    1. Dysgerminoma
    2. Theca cell tumor
    3. Hilus cell tumor
    4. Granulosa cell tumor

345. Membranous glomerulonephritis may be associated with
    1. hepatitis B infection
    2. lymphomas
    3. use of mercurial diuretics
    4. systemic lupus erythematosus

346. If the cervical Papanicolaou smear of a 21-year-old nulliparous woman shows cytologic evidence of cervical intraepithelial neoplasm, the currently accepted procedure include(s)
    1. cervical conization
    2. lesional localization through colposcopy
    3. four-quadrant cervical biopsy
    4. directed punch biopsy and endocervical curettage

347. Which of the following ovarian tumors arise(s) from the surface coelomic epithelium?
    1. Mucinous cystadenoma
    2. Choriocarcinoma
    3. Clear cell carcinoma
    4. Granulosa-theca cell tumors

		Directions Summarized		
A	B	C	D	E
1,2,3	1,3	2,4	4	All are
only	only	only	only	correct

348. Rapidly progressive glomerulonephritis
1. may arise as an immune complex disease
2. may arise as antiglomerular basement membrane (GMB) disease
3. characteristically produces a rapidly worsening renal function
4. produces proliferative glomerulonephritis with diffuse crescent formation

349. Membranoproliferative glomerulonephritis
1. may otherwise be called mesangiocapillary glomerulonephritis
2. commonly occurs in children and adolescents
3. morphologically shows a "double-contour" outline of glomerular capillaries
4. may show a striking depression of beta-1-C globulin

350. Which of the following renal lesions characterizes malignant hypertension?
1. Hyperplastic arteriolosclerosis
2. Hyaline arteriosclerosis
3. Necrotizing arteriolitis
4. Exudative lesions

351. The most common form of hereditary nephritis is
1. associated with nerve deafness
2. autosomal dominant
3. associated with the presence of foam cells in the interstitium
4. progressive only in males

352. Necrotizing papillitis may be found in
1. diabetes mellitus
2. Henoch-Schönlein syndrome
3. analgesic abuse
4. lupus nephritis

353. Concerning carcinoma of the penis, it may be said that
1. it is most common among Jews
2. about 10% are adenocarcinomas
3. it is extremely rare in noncircumcised Muslims
4. the lesion usually begins on the glans penis

354. The borderline group of serous or mucinous tumor of the ovary is identified by the
1. absence of complex papillary pattern
2. absence of cellular pleomorphism
3. complete loss of columnar orientation
4. absence of invasion

355. True statement(s) concerning cervical intraepithelial neoplasm (CIN) of the uterine cervix include(s) the following.
1. CIN grade 3 is synonymous with severe dysplasia and/or carcinoma in situ
2. Genital herpes virus type 2 is linked to the development of CIN
3. The lesion almost always begins at the squamo-columnar junction
4. On colposcopic examination, the presence of a mosaic or punctate pattern correlates with a histologic diagnosis of CIN

356. Lichen sclerosus of the vulva
1. clinically manifests plaquelike whitish pruritic lesion
2. is regarded by most investigators as definitely premalignant
3. histologically shows a thin epidermis with loss of rete ridges and collagenosis of the dermis
4. occurs most commonly in the third and fourth decades

Directions Summarized

A	B	C	D	E
1,2,3	1,3	2,4	4	All are
only	only	only	only	correct

357. The pathologic basis for the diagnosis of chronic endometritis depends on the presence of
1. epithelioid cells
2. lymphocytes
3. histiocytes
4. plasma cells

358. A high frequency of endometrial hyperplasia may be found in
1. prolonged anovulatory cycles
2. prolonged administration of estrogen
3. Stein-Leventhal syndrome
4. functioning granulosa-theca cell ovarian tumor

359. Young women whose mothers were treated with diethylstilbesterol (DES) have an increased incidence of
1. sarcoma bortyoides of the vagina
2. adenosis of the vagina
3. squamous cell carcinoma of the vagina
4. clear cell adenocarcinoma of the vagina

DIRECTIONS: Each group of questions below consists of five lettered headings followed by a list of numbered words, phrases, or statements. For **each** numbered word, phrase, or statement, select the **one** lettered heading that is most closely associated with it. Each lettered heading may be selected once, more than once, or not at all.

Questions 360–364:
- A. Goodpasture's syndrome
- B. Lipoid nephrosis
- C. Lupus nephritis
- D. Malignant hypertension
- E. Activation of the alternate complement pathway

360. Subendothelial immune deposit

361. Uniform flattening and loss of foot processes

362. Linear deposits of immunofluorescence

363. Type II membranoproliferative glomerulonephritis

364. Finely granular cortex with tiny petechial hemorrhages ("flea-bites")

Questions 365–371:
- A. Granulosa cell tumors
- B. Dysgerminomas
- C. Ovarian fibroma
- D. Endodermal sinus tumor
- E. Hilus cell tumor

365. Chorionic gonadotropin

366. Meigs' syndrome

367. Alpha-fetoprotein

368. Reinke crystalloids

369. Call-Exner bodies

370. Radiosensitive

371. Virilization

Questions 372–378:
- A. Gartner's duct cyst
- B. Vaginal endometriosis
- C. Vaginal adenosis
- D. Vaginal mucinous cyst
- E. Vaginal squamous epithelial inclusion cyst

372. Commonly occurs in episiotomy scars

373. Lateral vaginal wall

374. Dilated vestiges of mesonephric ducts

375. Paramesonephric duct origin

376. Intrauterine diethylstilbestrol exposure

377. Colposcopic identification of tiny foci of reddened velvety lesions

378. Clear cell adenocarcinoma

Questions 379–385:
- **A.** Adult polycystic kidney disease
- **B.** Childhood polycystic kidney disease
- **C.** Medullary sponge kidney
- **D.** Uremic medullary cystic disease complex
- **E.** None of the above

379. Associated with cystic disease of the liver in almost all cases

380. Cysts, lined by flattened epithelium, predominantly at the cortico-medullary junction

381. Nearly all are inherited as an autosomal dominant trait

382. Intracranial aneurysms

383. Secondary to maintenance hemodialysis

384. Though grossly cystic, histologically reveals immature ductules, undifferentiated mesenchyme, and cartilage

385. Benign, asymptomatic, and usually discovered as an incidental radiologic finding

Questions 386–392:
- A. Meckel's diverticulum
- B. Hirschsprung's disease
- C. Pyloric stenosis
- D. Cystic fibrosis
- E. Enteric cysts

386. Failure to find ganglion cells in adequate rectal biopsy

387. Surgical resection of narrowed and nonhypertrophied segment

388. Most common of many possible residua of omphalomesenteric duct

389. In 25% of cases, mucosa is of gastric type

390. Relief obtained by surgical incision of hypertrophied muscle

391. Commonly related to the esophagus

392. Meconium ileus

Questions 393–397:
- A. Galactosemia
- B. Erythroblastosis fetalis
- C. Phenylketonuria (PKU)
- D. Respiratory distress syndrome in the newborn (RDS)
- E. Cystic fibrosis (CF)

393. Musty or mouselike odor of untreated patients

394. Quantitative pilocarpine iontophoretic sweat test

395. Hepatosplenomegaly, cataracts, and hepatic failure

396. Edema of the brain with bright yellow pigmentation in the basal ganglia

397. Deficiency of lecithin phospholipid

DIRECTIONS: The set of lettered headings below is followed by a list of numbered words or phrases. For each numbered word or phrase select

A if the item is associated with (A) *only*

B if the item is associated with (B) *only*

C if the item is associated with *both* (A) *and* (B)

D if the item is associated with *neither* (A) *nor* (B)

Questions 398 – 402:

A. Ischemic acute tubular necrosis

B. Toxic acute tubular necrosis

C. Both

D. Neither

398. Proximal convoluted tubule most prominently affected

399. Flattened epithelial cells with hyperchromatic nuclei, binucleated cells, and mitosis

400. Tubular cells containing large acidophilic inclusions

401. Ruptured basement membrane (tubulorrhexis)

402. Reactive mesangial proliferation with capillary congestion

Answers and Comments

322. D. Malignant testicular tumors cause progressive painless enlargement of the testis. Choriocarcinoma may not be palpable but may be accompanied by gynecomastia, large amounts of chorionic gonadotropin in urine, and large mediastinal and pulmonary metastases. (REF. 5, p. 1170)

323. B. Diffuse glomerulosclerosis produces structural changes in the basement membrane over a much larger area than that seen with nodular glomerulosclerosis. Proteinuria with subsequent edema appears to be related to structural changes seen in the basement membrane. (REF. 2, p. 755)

324. C. The arterioles of the affected kidney are usually protected from the effects of hypertension caused by renal artery stenosis; by contrast, the arterioles of the contralateral kidney show hypertensive changes such as hyaline arteriosclerosis. (REF. 1, pp. 1047–1048)

325. A. Fanconi syndrome is a primary disorder of tubular function. Aminoaciduria and glycosuria may result owing to impairment of tubular absorptive function. The glomeruli do not show any primary changes in Fanconi syndrome. (REF. 1, pp. 408, 1009)

326. E. In myeloma of the kidney the glomeruli usually appear to be normal or may show minimal ischemic changes. The interstitium contains nonspecific inflammatory infiltrate. The most dramatic change is the presence of casts within the distal convoluted and collecting tubules. (REF. 1, p. 1040)

327. C. Within the group of membranoproliferative glomerulonephritis, dense deposit disease appears to be a distinctive clinical and pathologic entity. Ultrastructurally, the most striking feature is the presence of a dense linear deposit in the basement membrane. (REF. 1, p. 1017)

328. A. Option A refers to a lesion characteristically observed in myeloma of the kidney. In addition to the other listed lesions, systemic lupus erythematosus may cause necrotizing arteriolitis and arteritis in the kidney. Patients with focal glomerulonephritis have a uniformly good prognosis; those with membranous disease generally fare poorly. Renal failure in patients with systemic lupus erythematosus appears to be more closely related to the initial severity of the lesion. (REF. 1, p. 1021)

329. A. Pathologically, membranous nephropathy with its scattered subepithelial deposits (stage 1) is followed by the typical alteration of deposits and "spikes" (stages 2 and 3), which finally leads to a diffuse thickening of the basement membrane (stage 4). There is a rough correlation between the histologic stages and the duration of the disease. (REF. 1, p. 1012)

330. B. A very characteristic hydropic degeneration is observed in renal tubular epithelial cells in association with hypokalemia. The pathogenic mechanism of this change is not clear. (REF. 1, p. 1039)

331. E. Goodpasture's nephritis is an example of anti-GBM disease. The deposits seen by immunofluorescent techniques in the glomeruli are linear in configuration and can be seen in the basement membrane. (REF. 1, p. 1010)

332. D. Morphologic characteristics observed in Stein-Leventhal syndrome include multiple subcortical ovarian cysts and ovarian cortical hyperplasia. The clinical problems appear to be related to failure of ovulation. The presence of an involuted corpus luteum is inconsistent with this diagnosis. (REF. 1, p. 1142)

333. B. Von Hansemann cells are large histiocytes with granular cytoplasm containing Michaelis-Gutman bodies (MGB), which are identified by their small, rounded, and laminated configuration. MGB, which stain with iron, periodic-acid Schiff, and von Kossa stains, are believed to be breakdown products of bacteria or altered bacteria that become mineralized. (REF. 1, pp. 1069–1070)

334. C. Salpingitis isthmica nodosa is characterized by the presence of bilateral nodular enlargements of the tubal isthmi; the nodules may be multiple and vary from a few millimeters to a few centimeters. Although apparently acquired, the pathogenesis is unknown. Inflammatory changes are inconspicuous or absent, and most patients are sterile. (REF. 2, p. 1495)

335. D. Reinke crytalloids are rod-shaped intracytoplasmic inclusions found in about half of Leydig (interstitial) cell tumors. The tumor cells, which are large, have abundant cytoplasm as well as lipids, vacuoles and/or lipochrome pigment. (REF. 1, pp. 1097–1098)

336. C. Alpha-fetoprotein and alpha-1 antitrypsin can be demonstrated by immunocytochemical methods in the cytoplasm of endodermal sinus tumor cells as well as in extracellular eosinophilic hyaline globules which are commonly found in the tumor. (REF. 1, p. 1094)

337. B. In Berger's disease, deposits of IgA are found in the mesangium; additionally, C3, properdin, and lesser amounts of IgG or IgM may be present. (REF. 1, p. 1019)

338. A. Crescents result from proliferation of parietal epithelial cells, probably as a response to the leakage of fibrin from damaged glomerular walls. (REF. 1, p. 1011)

339. D. Evidence exists that implicates hyperestrenism or prolonged estrogen intake as predisposing to endometrial adenocarcinoma. Diabetes mellitus and hypertension are observed in 5%–11% and 5% of patients with endometrial adenocarcinoma respectively. (REF. 1, p. 1138)

340. D. Under the influence of estrogen and progesterone produced by the ovary, the endometrium undergoes cyclical changes. The changes occurring in the first half of the cycle, the proliferative phase, are under the influence of estrogen while progesterone and, to a lesser extent, estrogen, influence the changes of the latter half (secretory phase) of the menstrual cycle. The latter is heralded within 24 to 36 hours of ovulation by subnuclear vacuolation of endometrial glands. Subsequently, the secretory activity increases, the glands become more tortuous, and a variety of stromal and vascular changes ensue, leading finally to menstruation on the 28th day. (REF. 6, pp. 1110–1112)

341. A. Metastases from mucinous cystadenocarcinoma of the ovary to the peritoneum results in a diffuse gelatinous and mucinous material coating abdominal viscera. A similar lesion may result from the rupture of mucinous carcinoma of the appendix. (REF. 1, p. 1146)

342. D. The blood and urine of some patients with testicular germ cell tumors may contain large amounts of chorionic gonadotropin, follicle-stimulating, and other hormones, and alpha-fetoprotein. These substances, particularly gonadotropin and alpha-fetoprotein, may be used as tumor markers to assess the postoperative course of the patient. Pure choriocarcinoma is rare; more commonly, it occurs with other germ cell tumors, and in the latter setting, the prognosis is not as hopeless. (REF. 2, pp. 800–801)

343. C. Carcinoids of the gastrointestinal tract have not been associated with the classic carcinoid syndrome unless metastasis to the liver is present. In contrast, several cases of ovarian carcinoid present with the characteristic symptoms without hepatic metastasis. It is postulated that the difference in the venous drainage between the primary sites may account for the variations in symptomatology. (REF. 1, p. 845)

344. C. Estrogen-producing (feminizing) tumors of the ovary have been observed to coexist with endometrial carcinoma in a much higher ratio than the laws of chance would permit. Dysgerminomas are usually biologically inert; hilus cell tumors are generally virilizing. (REF. 1, p. 1138)

345. E. In most cases the pathogenesis of membranous glomerulonephritis is unknown; however, there is a growing list of drugs, heavy metals, infections, and tumors that have been found to be associated with this disease. (REF. 1, pp. 1013–1014)

346. C. Cervical intraepithelial neoplasm (CIN) is becoming very common in women in the 20s and early 30s. Preservation of the childbearing function in this age group is of paramount importance. Cervical conization has been associated with subsequent difficulties, either due to cervical stenosis or cervical incompetence. Following colposcopic lesional localization, directed punch biopsy, and endocervical curettage, electrocoagulation or cryotherapy may be performed, followed with Papanicolaou smears to rule out possible recurrence. Conization is reserved for a small percentage of patients whose lesions are not eradicated by electrocoagulation or cryotherapy. A still smaller percentage of these patients may require hysterectomy to remove foci of CIN not eradicated by conization. (REF. 1, pp. 1125–1128)

347. B. The surface coelomic epithelium has the potential of differentiating into epithelium that closely resembles the fallopian tubes (serous), the endometrial lining (endometrioid), or the endocervical glands (mucinous). Because clear cell adenocarcinoma resembles renal cell carcinoma, this ovarian tumor was presumed to originate from renal anlagen and was referred to as "mesonephroid." It is now thought that clear cell adenocarcinomas of the ovary arise from the coelomic epithelium. Choriocarcinoma is a germ cell tumor; granulosa-theca cell tumors originate from the ovarian stroma. (REF. 1, p. 1143)

348. E. Rapidly progressive glomerulonephritis does not appear to be a distinct immunologic entity. It can be considered as an ominous sequel of various forms of acute glomerulonephritis. (REF. 1, p. 1009)

349. E. The characteristic morphological appearances are those of capillary wall thickening and increased mesangial matrix and cellularity. The clinical picture is a mixture of acute nephritic and nephrotic features. Both hematuria and proteinuria are present. Hypocomplementemia principally affecting the C3 component but also C7 is usual in membranoproliferative glomerulonephritis which is a progressive disorder. While 78% of patients survive 5 years, only about 50% survive 10 years, and probably none survive 15 years after diagnosis. (REF. 1, p. 1016)

350. B. Hyperplastic arteriosclerosis is seen under the light microscope as onion-skin, concentric laminated thickening of the walls of arterioles. An immunologic reaction has been suggested as etiologic in the arteriolitis because complement and gammaglobulin are known to be located in arteriolar walls. (REF. 1, p. 1046)

351. E. The nephropathy usually appears in the first two decades of life, and most males die before the age of 40. The morphological renal changes are not distinctive. In some, proliferative glomerulitis may be present; in others glomerular basement membrane thickening is found. (REF. 1, p. 1026)

352. B. Necrotizing papillitis may also be associated with urinary tract obstruction. Its genesis is obscure, but it may be an expression of the vulnerability of the medulla to infection and of the peculiar pattern of blood supply to the pyramids. (REF. 1, p. 1032)

353. D. Circumcision appears to be protective against the development of squamous carcinoma of the penis. The accumulation of smegma with subsequent irritation and chronic inflammation in noncircumcised individuals seems to play a pathogenic role. Religious injunction calls for circumcision in early neonatal period among the Jews. Among Muslims, circumcision is generally performed at a later date during childhood. The protective effect of early circumcision among Jews appears to be related to the lower incidence of carcinoma of the penis in this group. (REF. 1, p. 1084)

354. D. The identification of borderline tumors is important, particularly in the management of young patients. Although of unpredictable behavior, as a group they have much better prognosis than do malignant ovarian tumors. The chief diagnostic feature of this tumor is the lack of invasion. Complex papillary pattern is often present. The moderately dysplastic cells still maintain their columnar orientation in some areas. (REF. 1, p. 1144)

355. E. High incidence of carcinoma of the cervix has been correlated with low socioeconomic status, early marriage and increased parity, frequency of coitus and age of onset of sexual relations, and viral infections such as herpes simplex, type 2, and human papilloma virus. (REF. 1, p. 1123)

356. B. Three types of vulvar dystrophy occur: lichen sclerosus (atrophic dystrophy), hypertrophic dystrophy, and mixed dystrophy in which a mixture of the two types coexist. Clinically, the lesion is usually pruritic and may be white, red, or a combination of both.

Malignant change has been shown to occur in about 1%–3% of patients. (REF. 2, pp. 1459–1461)

357. D. Lymphocytes, histiocytes, and neutrophils are found in normal menstrual endometrium. Additionally scattered lymphocytes are normally present throughout the menstrual cycle. (REF. 2, p. 1484; REF. 1, p. 1130)

358. E. The diagnostic terms used to describe endometrial hyperplasia are varied and sometimes confusing. Three types are recognized: cystic (mild), adenomatous (moderate), and atypical endometrial hyperplasia. All result from prolonged endogenous or exogenous estrogen stimulation with diminished or absent progesterone activity. (REF. 1, pp. 1133–1134; REF. 2, pp. 1484–1486)

359. C. In vaginal adenosis, there is focal replacement of squamous epithelium by Müllerian or columnar epithelium; the latter may also be found in the submucosa. This lesion, most probably, is a precursor of clear cell adenocarcinoma of the vagina. (REF. 1, pp. 1120–1121)

360. C. This electron-microscopic appearance is characteristic of acute proliferative lupus nephritis and is responsible for the "wire-loop" lesions seen by light microscopy. (REF. 1, p. 1022)

361. B. By light microscopy, lipoid nephrosis shows no glomerular basement or cellular changes. By immunofluorescence, deposition of immunoglobulins or complement is not demonstrable. (REF. 1, p. 1014)

362. A. The linear deposits are produced by antiglomerular basement membrane antibodies. In man, this mechanism of renal injury is much less common than the immune complex type. (REF. 1, p. 1010)

363. E. In type II membranoproliferative glomerulonephritis, there is deposition of electron-dense material in the lamina densa of the glomerular basement membrane transforming the latter into a thickened prominent electron dense structure — dense deposit disease. By immunofluorescence, C3 is usually demonstrated in irregular granular-linear foci within the glomerular basement membrane while IgG is often absent and the early acting complement components (C1q and C4) are always absent. (REF. 1, p. 1016)

364. D. The gross morphology of the kidney in malignant hypertension (in this case secondary to preexisting chronic glomerulonephritis) reflects glomerular sclerosis, tubular atrophy, interstitial fibrosis, and thrombonecrotic glomerular and vascular lesions. (REF. 1, p. 1046)

365. B. Some dysgerminomas produce human chorionic gonadotropin (HCG). This hormone may be used as a tumor marker for evaluation of the patient's posttherapy course. (REF. 2, p. 1512)

366. C. Fibromas, also referred to as burnt-out thecomas, are densely collagenized fibrous tumors that lack endocrine activity, and they may occasionally be associated with benign ascites and pleural effusion; this triad constitutes Meigs' syndrome. The effusions disappear after resection of the tumor. (REF. 2, p. 1510)

367. D. Alpha-fetoprotein is normally produced in the yolk sac and liver of a developing embryo. Endodermal sinus tumor, a rare tumor that develops through extraembryonal differentiation of germ cells, consistently produces this substance. This protein may be used as a tumor marker for early detection of recurrence. (REF. 2, p. 1512)

368. E. Like Leydig cells of the testis, ovarian hilus cells may contain eosinophilic, slender rodlike cytoplasmic inclusions or bodies with rounded, tapering, or square ends, measuring 10 and 20 μ in length (Reinke crystalloids). These bodies, which are better visualized with Masson's trichrome-stained section, are specific enough to allow differentiation from other types of "lipoid cells." (REF. 2, p. 1511)

369. A. Call-Exner bodies are almost always present in granulosa cell tumors. These bodies consist of rounded masses of pink inspissated material surrounded by a circular row of granulosa cells which produces the characteristic rosettelike structures. (REF. 2, p. 1509)

370. B. Dysgerminoma is extremely radiosensitive; the basic treatment would therefore be surgical excision followed by radiotherapy, the extent of which depends upon tumor spread and distribution of metastases. Many cases are radiocurable even in the presence of metastases. (REF. 2, p. 1512)

371. E. The adult ovarian hilus contains cell nests that are morphologically identical with testicular Leydig cells. Like the latter, these are androgenic in function. Virilization is the most common endocrine abnormality. (REF. 2, p. 1510)

372. B. Vaginal endometriosis forms multiple blue mucosal cysts usually caused by implantation of endometrium in an incision, particularly an episiotomy. These foci may rupture and bleed during menses. (REF. 1, p. 1130)

373. A. Gartner's cysts of the anterolateral or lateral vaginal wall are considered to arise from dilated vestiges of mesonephric ducts and are lined by cuboidal epithelium. Cytoplasmic mucin is absent in these cells. (REF. 2, p. 1119)

374. A. See explanatory answer 378. (REF. 2, p. 1669)

375. D. Mucinous cysts appear to be more commonly situated near the vestibule and are considered to be of paramesonephric duct origin. (REF. 2, p. 1468)

376. C. In adenosis, benign mucinous epithelium of typical endocervical pattern is present in areas normally covered by opaque, pale pink, stratified squamous epithelium. The lesions are reddish and velvety, ranging from tiny foci of 1 to 2 mm in diameter to extensive lesions involving the entire vaginal lining. Tiny focal lesions require colposcopic examination for identification. Causal relationship with intrauterine diethylstilbestrol exposure has been demonstrated; the crucial period of fetal exposure is prior to the eighteenth week of gestation. Both the clear cell adenocarcinomas and the mucinous epithelium of adenosis are most probably of Müllerian duct origin. (REF. 2, p. 1468)

377. C. See explanatory answer 376. (REF. 2, p. 1468)

378. C. Clear cell adenocarcinomas associated with adenosis in adolescent girls with intrauterine exposure to diethylstilbestrol or its derivatives have histologic patterns identical to those of clear cell carcinomas occurring elsewhere in the body. (REF. 3, p. 1468; REF. 5, p. 1286)

379. B. Some patients with childhood polycystic disease may also develop congenital hepatic fibrosis, a disease characterized by portal fibrosis and proliferated bile ducts. This lesion has also been reported in some patients with adult polycystic disease, one third of whom may also have polycystic liver disease. (REF. 1, pp. 1000–1001)

380. D. In addition to medullary cysts, nephronophthisis-medullary cystic disease complex shows cortical tubular atrophy and interstitial fibrosis. Progressive renal failure is the rule and death ensues 5 to 10 years after the onset of symptoms. Clinically patients have anemia, salt-losing syndrome, tubular concentration defect, and azotemia. (REF. 2, p. 767)

381. A. Not only is the inheritance of adult polycystic kidney disease dominant, the penetrance is high, approximating 100% in patients who survive to their eighth and ninth decades. (REF. 1, p. 1000)

382. A. Berry aneurysms of the circle of Willis occur in about 15% of patients with adult polycystic kidney disease. Other anomalies that may be encountered include cysts of the liver, pancreas, and lungs. (REF. 1, p. 1000)

383. E. The kidneys of patients on long-term maintenance hemodialysis may show acquired cortical and medullary cysts ranging from 0.5 to 2 cm in dimension. These lesions may be complicated by benign epithelial renal tumors and renal oxalosis. (REF. 1, p. 1002)

384. E. These features accurately describe cystic renal dysplasia, a sporadic disorder associated with obstructive abnormalities of the ureter and lower urinary tract. (REF. 1, pp. 999–1000)

385. C. Medullary sponge kidney, though benign, may be complicated by pyelonephritis and calculi formation. (REF. 1, p. 1001)

386. B. Also known as aganglionic megacolon, this disease is characterized by symptoms of complete or partial intestinal obstruction usually occurring at birth or early in life. The lack of ganglion cells in Auerbach's (myenteric) and Meissner's (submucous) plexuses is the basic defect. The aganglionic segment is narrowed but not hypertrophied. Conversely, the normally innervated intestine proximal to this area is markedly dilated and hypertrophied. Surgical resection of the aganglionic segment relieves the condition. (REF. 1, p. 855)

387. B. See explanatory answer 386. (REF. 1, p. 855)

388. A. Other omphalomesenteric-duct residua include umbilical sinus, cyst between ileum and umbilicus, and ileoumbilical fistula. Gastric mucosa, when present (25% of cases), may result in peptic ulceration and hemorrhage. The majority of the diverticula have small intestinal mucosa. (REF. 1, p. 830)

389. A. See explanatory answer 388. (REF. 1, p. 830)

390. C. The etiology of the hypertrophy of the pyloric muscle that produces pyloric narrowing, is unknown. This condition is usually seen in male infants, producing vomiting with resultant dehydration and malnutrition. Surgical incision of the hypertrophied muscle gives relief. (REF. 1, p. 855)

391. E. Enteric cysts are segments of the gastrointestinal tube that are spherical and lack communication with the gut lumen. These are often intrathoracic and related to the esophagus. They may be lined by gastric, small intestinal, or bronchial mucosa. (REF. 2, pp. 1055–1056)

392. D. Intestinal obstruction occurs during the newborn period in 12%–15% of patients with cystic fibrosis. The obstructing lesion is a plug of chalky inspissated meconium in the distal ileum. Ileal atresia, volvulus, or perforation, with meconium peritonitis, may occur secondarily. The occurrence of this type of ileus correlates more with dilatation of intestinal glands by inspissated mucus secretions than with the severity of pancreatic lesions. (REF. 1, pp. 493 – 495)

393. C. Blood phenylalanine levels progressively rise in untreated patients with classic PKU because the hepatic phenylalanine-hydroxylase needed for the conversion of phenylalanine to tyrosine is absent. Phenylalanine appears in the urine when the serum level reaches 25–30 mg/dl. Eventually its abnormal metabolites (phenylpyruvic acid, ortho-hydroxyphenylacetic acid, and phenylacetic acid) are also excreted in the urine. The peculiar musty or mousey odor of untreated patients has been attributed to the phenylacetic acid. (REF. 1, pp. 490–491)

394. E. CF is very common and frequently fatal in childhood and young adult life. Although the etiology of the disease is unknown, it is basically a disorder of exocrine glands affecting both eccrine sweat glands and mucus-secreting glands throughout the body. Early diagnosis and, thus, proper management significantly prolong survival. The most reliable tool is a carefully performed quantitative pilocarpine iontophoretic sweat test. This test should be interpreted by an experienced physician and should be carried out in duplicate, or repeated at least once. A positive sweat test should be correlated with the clinical findings. (REF. 1, pp. 493–495)

395. A. Galactosemia results from a hereditary (autosomal recessive) deficiency of an enzyme involved in galactose metabolism. Two forms are identified: (1) galactose-1-phosphate uridyl transferase deficiency and (2) galactokinase deficiency (relatively benign). In the classic pattern, characterized by total absence of transferase, galactose cannot be metabolized to carbon dioxide. Infants with untreated homozygous disease appear normal at birth but soon after milk feeding develop listlessness, vomiting, diarrhea, and failure to thrive. Jaundice appears early and is soon followed by hepatosplenomegaly, cataracts, and signs of hepatic failure and death in early infancy. Progressive mental retardation is also one of the characteristic features of this disorder. Diagnosis is readily established through a variety of tests, such as: (1) determination of serum and urine galactose levels and (2) determination of transferase in cultured fibroblasts derived from amniotic fluid. (REF. 1, pp. 491–493)

396. B. In severe hemolytic disease bilirubin rises rapidly within the first day of life to reach extremely high levels (>20 mg/dl). Low-birth-weight and premature infants are at greatest risk because their conjugating and excretory systems cannot handle the bilirubin overload. Unconjugated bilirubin is water-soluble and has an affinity for lipids. In the infant with poorly developed blood-brain barrier, the unconjugated bilirubin (particularly toxic to the brain) may bind with the brain lipid and produce serious damage. The brain is edematous, and has a bright yellow pigmentation (kernicterus) particularly in the basal ganglia, thalamus, cerebellum, cerebral gray matter, and spinal cord. (REF. 1, pp. 486–490)

397. D. The fundamental defect of RDS is a deficiency of lecithin phospholipid (pulmonary surfactant). With normal levels of surfactant the lungs retain 40% of the residual air volume after the first breath, thus subsequent breaths require much lower inspiratory pressures. Lungs collapse when the surfactant is deficient and the infant must work as hard with each successive breath as it did with the first. (REF. 1, pp. 482–485)

398. B. The distal tubular segments are spared in nephrotoxic acute tubular necrosis (ATN). Ischemic ATN is characterized by mild focal tubular necrosis along the nephron often accompanied by tubulorrhexis. (REF. 1, p. 1027)

399. C. This is the morphologic expression of regeneration secondary to tubular necrosis. These changes are usually subtle and may be difficult to identify. Rarely, multinucleated renal epithelial cells are found. (REF. 1, p. 1027)

400. B. In some cases nephrotoxic ATN may show distinctive features that reveal possible etiologies. For example, ATN in ethylene glycol poisoning shows ballooning and hydropic degeneration associated with intraluminal deposit of calcium oxalate crystals. Tubular cells containing large acidophilic inclusions are seen in mercuric chloride toxicity. (REF. 1, pp. 1027–1028)

401. A. This feature distinguishes ischemic ATN from nephrotoxic ATN. Additionally, the distal tubular segments are usually unaffected by nephrotoxic ATN. (REF. 1, p. 1027)

402. D. The glomeruli are spared in acute tubular necrosis although fibrin deposition and platelet thrombi have been reported in some cases. (REF. 1, p. 1028)

7 Hematopoietic System

DIRECTIONS: Each of the questions or incomplete statements below is followed by five suggested answers or completions. Select the **one** that is best in each case.

---

403. The combination of calvarial bone defects, diabetes insipidus, and exophthalmos is strongly suggestive of
    A. Hand-Schuller-Christian disease (multifocal eosinophilic granuloma
    B. Letterer-Siwe disease (progressive differentiated histiocytosis)
    C. eosinophilic granuloma
    D. histiocytic medullary reticulosis
    E. multiple myeloma

404. Which of the following is LEAST likely to be encountered in nonspecific acute splenitis?
    A. Enlarged, soft, and frequently diffluent spleen
    B. Reticuloendothelial hyperplasia
    C. Gandy-Gamna bodies
    D. Necrosis of splenic lymphoid follicles
    E. Infiltration of neutrophils, plasma cells, and occasionally eosinophils

405. Chloromas are typically associated with
    A. myelogenous leukemia
    B. lymphatic leukemia
    C. myelomonocytic leukemia
    D. follicular lymphoma
    E. diffuse lymphoma

406. In an enlarged cervical lymph node associated with acute tonsillitis, the LEAST likely pathologic change that may be observed is
    A. prominence of lymphoid follicles
    B. large germinal centers
    C. striking increase in the number of immunoblasts
    D. histiocytes containing particulate debris
    E. necrosis with neutrophilic exudate

407. Which of the following features is NOT typically found in pernicious anemia?
    A. "Intestinalization" of gastric mucosa
    B. Atrophic glossitis
    C. Megaloblastic bone marrow
    D. An increased excretion of formiminoglutamic acid following a dose of histidine
    E. Posterolateral degeneration of the spinal cord

408. Serum haptoglobin level is a useful test for the diagnosis of anemia caused by
    A. acute blood loss
    B. intravascular hemolysis
    C. chronic infection
    D. arthritis
    E. malignancy

409. In microangiopathic hemolytic anemia, trauma to the red cell produces all of the following abnormalities EXCEPT
    A. schistocytes
    B. triangle cells
    C. Pelger cells
    D. burr cells
    E. helmet cells

410. Microangiopathic hemolytic anemia is characterized by all of the following EXCEPT
  A. macrocytic nonmegaloblastic anemia
  B. association with hemolytic uremic syndrome
  C. presence of schistocytes in the peripheral blood
  D. association with thrombotic thrombocytopenic purpura
  E. association with systemic lupus erythematosus

411. Macrocytosis may NOT be seen in association with
  A. anemia of pregnancy
  B. pernicious anemia
  C. folic acid deficiency anemia
  D. hemolytic anemia associated with pyruvate kinase deficiency
  E. anemia of *Diphyllobothrium latum* infestation

412. Coombs' positive autoimmune hemolytic anemia is LEAST likely to occur as a secondary manifestation of
  A. collagen vascular diseases
  B. lymphomas
  C. sarcoidosis
  D. infectious mononucleosis
  E. feto-maternal hemorrhage

413. A malignant lymphoma, common in women, and with a striking propensity to occur in the mediastinum, supraclavicular, and lower cervical nodes, is most likely to be
  A. Hodgkin's disease, nodular sclerosis type
  B. Burkitt's lymphoma
  C. Hodgkin's disease, lymphocyte predominant type
  D. nodular lymphoma, intermediate cell type
  E. Hodgkin's disease, lymphocyte depletion type

DIRECTIONS: For each of the questions or incomplete statements below, **one** or **more** of the answers or completions given is correct. Select

  A if only *1, 2, and 3* are correct
  B if only *1 and 3* are correct
  C if only *2 and 4* are correct
  D if only *4* is correct
  E if all are correct

---

414. Retroviruses have been implicated as etiologic agents in
    1. Hodgkin's disease, lymphocyte predominant type
    2. T-cell leukemia endemic in Japan and the Caribbean
    3. Burkitt's lymphoma
    4. acquired immune deficiency syndrome

415. The lacunar type of Reed Sternberg (RS) cell is found in which type(s) of Hodgkin's disease?
    1. Lymphocyte predominant
    2. Mixed cellularity
    3. Lymphocyte depletion
    4. Nodular sclerosis

416. Disseminated intravascular coagulation (DIC) is characterized by
    1. consumption of fibrinogen and prothrombin
    2. hemorrhagic diathesis
    3. diminished serum concentrations for factors V, VIII, and X
    4. formation of thrombi in large vessels

417. Monoclonal gammopathy is an important characteristic feature of
    1. gamma-chain disease
    2. μ-chain disease
    3. alpha-chain disease
    4. Waldenström's macroglobulinemia

418. Sickle cell nephropathy is characterized by
   1. diminished concentrating ability
   2. vascular occlusion of small intrarenal vessels
   3. papillary necrosis
   4. hematuria

419. Which of the following features are typical of beta-thalassemia major?
   1. Suppression of the beta chain of hemoglobin A
   2. Hypochromic, microcytic anemia
   3. Erythrocytes containing Heinz bodies
   4. Schizocytes ("helmet" cells)

420. Long-standing polycythemia vera may result in
   1. chronic myelogenous leukemia
   2. myelofibrosis
   3. erythroleukemia (Di Guglielmo's syndrome)
   4. anemia

421. A tentative separation of vitamin B_{12} deficiency from folic acid deficiency may be achieved by the presence of
   1. megaloblasts in the bone marrow
   2. high serum iron level
   3. elevated serum total iron-binding capacity
   4. hypersegmented neutrophils

422. A sharp spike in the gamma-globulin region on a plasma protein electrophoretic pattern would be seen but only on extremely rare occasions in which of the following diseases?
   1. Macroglobulinemia
   2. Franklin's disease
   3. Multiple myeloma
   4. Colonic adenocarcinoma

423. Abnormal globulins with peculiar property of precipitation when exposed to cold temperatures are seen in
   1. myeloma
   2. lymphoproliferative disorders
   3. Waldenström's disease
   4. systemic lupus erythematosus

Directions Summarized

A	B	C	D	E
1,2,3	1,3	2,4	4	All are
only	only	only	only	correct

424. The increase in the red cell mass seen in polycythemia vera is due to
    1. low oxygen tension of arterial blood supplying marrow
    2. a primary disorder of erythropoietic synthesis
    3. longer half-life of red cells
    4. apparent autonomy of erythropoietic mechanism

425. Hemolytic anemia has been associated with the deficiency state of which of the following enzymes?
    1. Pyruvate kinase
    2. Glutathione synthetase
    3. Triose-phosphate-isomerase
    4. 6-Phosphofructokinase

426. Low counts of peripheral blood elements in clinical hypersplenism may be related to
    1. the presence of specific antibodies against blood elements
    2. reticuloendothelial hyperplasia with enhanced phagocytosis
    3. substances elaborated by spleen capable of depression of marrow function or inhibition of release of cells from marrow
    4. sinusoidal proliferation and enlargement with diffuse thrombosis in spleen

DIRECTIONS: The group of questions below consists of five lettered headings followed by a list of numbered words, phrases, or statements. For **each** numbered word, phrase, or statement, select the **one** lettered heading that is most closely associated with it. Each lettered heading may be selected once, more than once, or not at all.

Questions 427–433:
- **A.** Acute myelomonocytic leukemia
- **B.** Chronic lymphatic leukemia (CLL)
- **C.** Chronic myelogenous leukemia (CML)
- **D.** Acute lymphoblastic leukemia (ALL)
- **E.** Hairy cell leukemia

427. Frequently associated with T-cell mediastinal lymphoma of childhood

428. Most striking splenomegaly

429. All forms of this leukemia show the presence of high concentration of terminal deoxynucleotidyl transferase

430. Most striking lymphadenopathy

431. Most likely to show Auer rods or bodies

432. Splenomegaly with lymphadenopathy, neutropenia, and thrombocytopenia

433. Philadelphia chromosome

DIRECTIONS: Each set of lettered headings below is followed by a list of numbered words or phrases. For each numbered word or phrase select
- **A** if the item is associated with (A) *only*
- **B** if the item is associated with (B) *only*
- **C** if the item is associated with *both* (A) *and* (B)
- **D** if the item is associated with *neither* (A) *nor* (B)

Questions 434 – 440:
- **A.** Extravascular hemolysis
- **B.** Intravascular hemolysis
- **C.** Both
- **D.** Neither

434. Microangiopathic hemolytic anemia

435. Schistocytes ("helmet" cells)

436. Glucose-6-phosphatase deficiency

437. Extramedullary hematopoicsis

438. Macrocytic erythrocytes and megaloblastic marrow

439. Hereditary spherocytosis

440. Diminished to absent marrow iron

Questions 441 – 447:
    A. T-cell derivation
    B. B-cell derivation
    C. Both
    D. Neither

441. Sézary syndrome

442. Burkitt's lymphoma

443. Follicular center cell lymphoma

444. Mycosis fungoides

445. Lymphoma with cerebriform nuclei

446. Most nodular lymphomas

447. Immunoblastic sarcoma

Answers and Comments

403. A. Patients with Hand-Schuller-Christian disease have fever, a diffuse scaly seborrheiclike eruption, mild lymphadenopathy, and hepatosplenomegaly. Orbital granulomas induce exophthalmos in about one-third of the patients and involvement of the posterior pituitary causes diabetes insipidus. (REF. 1, p. 694)

404. C. Gandy-Gamna bodies (nodules) found in congestive splenomegaly, are composed of foci of fibrosis containing deposits of iron and calcium salts encrusted on connective tissue and elastic fibers. (REF. 1, p. 701)

405. A. Chloromas are tumorous masses of myelogenous leukemia which may be found within soft tissues and any part of the skeleton but most often the skull. The tumors show an evanescent green color when first examined. (REF. 1, pp. 679–680)

406. C. Lymph nodes draining foci of acute inflammation show nonspecific acute lymphadenitis. Proliferation of immunoblasts and sinus histiocytosis are usually features found in chronic nonspecific reactive hyperplasia. Chronically inflamed lymph nodes are usually rubbery and nontender. (REF. 1, p. 656)

407. D. A number of immunologic derangements are associated with pernicious anemia. Antibodies are demonstrable in the serum of most patients with this disease of which the following are well recognized: "blocking" antibody which blocks vitamin B_{12}-intrinsic factor binding, "binding" antibody which reacts with intrinsic factor or intrinsic factor-B_{12} complex, and parietal canalicular antibody found in the microvilli of the canalicular system of the gastric parietal cell. (REF. 1, pp. 633–634)

408. B. Intravascular hemolysis results in the presence of free hemoglobin in the plasma. The haptoglobin combines with hemoglobin, and as a result the serum haptoglobin level falls. (REF. 3, p. 210)

409. C. Pelger cell refers to a leukocyte with a band-shaped nucleus. (REF. 3, p. 608)

410. A. Microangiopathic hemolytic anemia has been thought to result from damage to red cells initiated by vascular lesions. This is frequently seen as a part of the total picture of thrombocytopenic purpura, hemolytic uremic syndrome, renal cortical necrosis, and disseminated carcinoma. (REF. 3, p. 691)

411. D. *Diphyllobothrium latum* infestation appears to produce anemia by interfering with the absorption of vitamin B_{12}. Similar pathogenic mechanisms seem to play a role in the macrocytic anemias of pregnancy and infancy. (REF. 3, p. 657)

412. E. Coombs' positive autoimmune hemolytic anemia has been observed in association with all of the options in this question except feto-maternal hemorrhage. The diagnosis of idiopathic autoimmune hemolytic disease is often made by a process of elimination. At times, the diagnosis of either idiopathic or secondary autoimmune hemolytic anemia can be established only after a prolonged period of observation and repeated examinations. (REF. 3, pp. 692–695)

413. A. The morphology of nodular sclerosis Hodgkin's disease is distinctive in two regards: the presence of bands of fibrocollagenous tissue which traverse and divide the lymph node into nodules of lymphoid tissue and lacunar Reed Sternberg cells. (REF. 1, pp. 670–671)

414. C. Human T-cell leukemia lymphoma virus (HTLV) is a newly recognized T virus which has been isolated from T-cell malignancies, most consistently from T-cell leukemia, endemic in certain parts of Japan and the Caribbean. Antibodies to HTLV-III (HIV) are commonly found in the sera of patients with AIDS and is presently being employed as a screening test for this disease. (REF. 1, p. 678; REF. 4, p. 486)

415. D. The lacunar RS cell contains a large hyperlobated nucleus with conspicuous reddish nucleolus and abundant cytoplasm. A clear space exists around the cell (thus the designation lacunar RS) probably due to artefactual retraction during fixation and processing of the tissue. (REF. 1, p. 671)

416. A. In DIC, fibrin thrombi are found in small vessels of many organs, especially the brain, kidneys, lungs, heart, adrenals, spleen, and liver. They may cause microinfarcts in the brain or focal tubular necrosis in the kidneys. (REF. 1, pp. 649–651)

417. E. Gamma-chain disease, encountered in the elderly, resembles a malignant lymphoma and is manifested by splenomegaly, hepatomegaly, lymphadenopathy, anemia, and fever. The patients are susceptible to infection and the clinical course may be rapidly downhill, death ensuing within a few months. Alpha-chain disease occurs predominantly in children and is characterized by lymphoid infiltration of the gastrointestinal and/or respiratory tract. (REF. 1, p. 693)

418. E. Proteinuria may also occur in up to 30% of sickle cell anemia patients. Focal occlusion of the vasa recta may be demonstrated by postmortem angiographic studies of the kidney. (REF. 1, pp. 620, 1049)

419. A. The thalassemia syndromes are characterized by diminished synthesis of the alpha or beta chain of hemoglobin A consequent to the relative excessive synthesis of the other chain. The disease is inherited as an autosomal condition. The heterozygous individual with a mild hematologic disorder is said to have thalassemia minor (thalassemia trait) while one with homozygous condition associated with a more serious clinical derangement is said to have thalassemia major. (REF. 1, pp. 624–625)

420. E. The concept of myeloproliferative diseases postulates that one or more cell lines originating in the bone marrow may proliferate abnormally or become neoplastic and that the particular cell line may change with time. Polycythemia vera is the prototype of myeloproliferative disease. Others include erythroleukemia, chronic granulocytic leukemia, megakaryocytic myelosis, and primary thrombocythemia. (REF. 1, p. 641)

421. D. Large polymorphonuclear cells with hypersegmentation of nuclei are generally seen in vitamin B_{12} deficiency. (REF. 1, pp. 633–635)

422. D. Multiple myeloma, macroglobulinemia, and Franklin's disease almost always show sharp spikes in the gamma globulin region. Nonlymphoid malignant neoplasms such as colonic carcinoma, has also demonstrated a spike in gamma globulin region, but only in a few documented cases. (REF. 3, p. 743)

423. E. Cryoglobulins have been seen in a variety of lymphoproliferative processes and plasma cell dyscrasias. In addition, they have been demonstrated in autoimmune disorders and appear to be mixes of autoantigens, autoantibodies, and cofactors. (REF. 3, pp. 933–934)

424. D. Extensive work has failed to show any increase in the half-life of red cells or bone marrow hypoxia in polycythemia vera. Erythropoietic metabolism also has not been shown to be abnormal in this condition. The etiology of polycythemia vera remains obscure and appears to be a phenomenon akin to a neoplastic process. (REF. 1, p. 641)

425. A. The deficiency states of the first three enzymes are rare disorders but have been known to produce clinical hemolytic anemia. The fourth enzyme—6-phosphofructokinase—deficiency is associated with a glycogen storage disorder. (REF. 1, p. 617; REF. 3, pp. 278 279)

426. A. The evidence for a low-grade intrasinusoidal thrombosis and destruction of blood elements in the form of fibrin thrombi in the sinusoids has not been documented. There is some evidence that seems to point to the existence of the first three mechanisms. (REF. 1, p. 699)

427. D. The L_1 type of ALL is at present thought to represent a T-cell disorder in which convoluted lymphocytes predominate. The L_3 pattern of ALL may be associated with Burkitt's lymphoma. (REF. 1, p. 675)

428. C. Splenic weights of 5 kg are not unusual in CML. Infarcts due to leukemic infiltration and obstruction of vessels are frequent. (REF. 1, p. 680)

429. D. Most cells of ALL are of the "null" type—unassociated with either B- or T-cell markers; cells from virtually all forms of ALL, however, have high concentrations of terminal deoxynucleotidyl transferase. (REF. 1, p. 676)

430. B. Lymph nodes throughout the body are usually enlarged in all forms of leukemia. While they are most prominently enlarged in CLL, they are only moderately or minimally enlarged in monocytic leukemia. (REF. 1, p. 687)

431. A. Auer rods, which are abnormal lysosomal structures, are found in myeloblasts and promyelocytes and less commonly in monocytic cells. (REF. 1, p. 679)

432. E. Hairy cell leukemia, otherwise called leukemic reticuloendotheliosis, is characterized by the appearance of "hairy cells" in the blood and bone marrow. Many cells are covered by innumerable villous projections, others have ridges and broad-based ruffles. The cells may originate from B lymphocytes or histiocytes. (REF. 1, p. 685)

433. C. In approximately 90% of patients with CML, Philadelphia chromosomes can be identified in myeloblasts, erythroblasts, and megakaryoblasts. The chromosome represents a translocation from chromosome 22 to chromosome 9. (REF. 1, p. 676)

434. B. Normal erythrocytes may be damaged by the shear stress imposed by thrombi within the microcirculation (disseminated intravascular coagulation) resulting in intravascular hemolysis—microangiopathic hemolytic anemia. (REF. 3, pp. 608, 691)

435. B. These cells which occur in abnormal shapes are the result of mechanical injury to the erythrocytes such as that caused by prosthetic cardiac ball valves, or disseminated intravascular coagulation. (REF. 3, p. 608)

436. A. Deficiency of erythrocytic glucose-6-phosphatase, an enzyme involving the hexose monophosphate shunt pathway, is a hereditary condition, which may lead to clinically significant hemolysis. Scores of genetic variants occur but only a few are known to cause significant hemolysis. (REF. 3, p. 279)

437. C. Other features of hemolytic anemias, regardless of their etiology, are reticulocytosis, active marrow with normoblastic hyperplasia, and elevated levels of bilirubin. (REF. 1, p. 615)

438. D. These are features of anemias caused by vitamin B_{12} and folic acid deficiency. (REF. 1, p. 633)

439. A. Hereditary spherocytosis is characterized by an intracorpuscular defect which renders the erythrocytes spheroidal and thus more susceptible to splenic sequestration and destruction. Splenectomy is curative in most cases. (REF. 1, p. 616)

440. D. These features are typical of iron deficiency anemia. (REF. 1, p. 638)

441. A. In Sezary's syndrome, there is infiltration of upper dermis and epidermis by lymphomatous cells with characteristics of T cells. The nuclei of the tumor cells are convoluted and cerebriform; sometimes they may be admixed with "histiocytes." The cells frequently spill into the blood producing a leukemic picture. (REF. 1, p. 665)

442. B. Burkitt's lymphoma is a diffuse extranodal lymphoma of undifferentiated cells with round to oval nuclei, prominent nucleoli and moderate amount of faintly basophilic cytoplasm. Scattered throughout the tumor are large phagocytes with abundant cytoplasm producing clear spaces, creating the characteristic "starry sky" appearance. The African type is strongly associated with Epstein-Barr virus infection. (REF. 1, p. 662)

443. B. These tumors may be composed of small or large cells with or without cleaved nuclei. In a normal follicle center, the noncleaved cells have the ability to divide while the cleaved cells are nondividing. (REF. 1, p. 663)

444. A. Sezary's syndrome and mycosis fungoides are related disorders with overlapping morphologic features. Unlike Sezary's syndrome, mycosis fungoides is generally not associated with a leukemic phase; skin infiltration with tumor formation is quite common in the late stages of mycosis fungoides. (REF. 1, p. 665)

445. A. These cells can be distinguished from small cleaved cells of B origin by the use of cell markers. (REF. 1, p. 665)

446. B. These lymphomas arise from the follicle center cell. Some however may be of the diffuse type, particularly in those composed of noncleaved cells. (REF. 1, p. 664)

447. C. Both immunoblastic sarcoma of B- and T-cell origin resemble each other morphologically; cell markers, however, permit their separation. (REF. 1, p. 664)

8 Endocrine System

448. A cystic lesion that is located in the midline near the hyoid bone is most likely to be
   A. ectopic parathyroid
   B. branchial cleft cyst
   C. throglossal duct cyst
   D. ectopic salivary gland tissue
   E. none of the above

449. Medullary carcinoma of the thyroid has been shown to secrete all of the following EXCEPT
   A. thyrocalcitonin
   B. adrenocorticotropic hormone
   C. prostaglandin
   D. histaminase
   E. thyroxine

450. Carcinoma of the thyroid is characterized by all of the following EXCEPT
  A. nearly half of the thyroid nodules in children are malignant
  B. a history of previous irradiation in infancy can be elicited in about 25% of patients
  C. the incidence is higher in girls than boys
  D. the tumor may be multifocal
  E. a follicular pattern is the predominant histologic type

451. All of these are true of adenoma of the anterior pituitary gland EXCEPT
  A. patients may show bilateral homonymous hemianopsia
  B. histological demonstration of Crooke's hyalin degeneration
  C. the most common endocrinopathy is the excessive production of growth hormone causing gigantism or acromegaly
  D. hypopituitarism may ensue in up to 25% of affected patients
  E. many of the small adenomas are unencapsulated

452. The measurement of which of the following analytes provides the most useful means of evaluating satisfactory long-term control of diabetes mellitus?
  A. Plasma glucose
  B. Serum glucose
  C. Two-hour postprandial plasma glucose
  D. HbA_{1c} (glycosylated hemoglobin)
  E. Two-hour glucose tolerance test

453. All of these are true of pancreatic pseudocysts EXCEPT
  A. they may be found within the pancreatic tissue but more often are located adjacent to the pancreas
  B. most are secondary to pancreatitis, pancreatic necrosis, or hemorrhage
  C. they usually are connected to the pancreatic duct system
  D. they are devoid of an epithelial lining
  E. they are usually unilocular

454. The current proposed pathogenesis of Graves' disease implicates
  A. dyshormogenesis
  B. granulomatous inflammation
  C. nonspecific chronic inflammation
  D. autoimmunity
  E. excessive production of thyroid-stimulating hormone

455. The autoantibody most commonly observed in patients with Hashimoto's thyroiditis is
  A. antithyroglobulin antibodies
  B. thyroid-stimulating immunoglobulin
  C. antimicrosomal antibodies
  D. thyroid-growth immunoglobulin
  E. T-suppressor cell antibody

DIRECTIONS: For each of the questions or incomplete statements below, **one** or **more** of the answers or completions given is correct. Select

  A if only *1, 2, and 3* are correct
  B if only *1 and 3* are correct
  C if only *2 and 4* are correct
  D if only *4* is correct
  E if all are correct

---

456. In which variant(s) of congenital hyperplasia of the adrenal cortex is 21-hydroxylase the enzymatic deficiency?
  1. Hypertensive form
  2. Simple virilizing forms
  3. Adrenal cortical lipid hyperplasia
  4. Salt-losing form

457. Somatostatin
  1. is derived from D (delta) cells of the islets of Langerhans
  2. inhibits thyrotropin, gastrin, and secretin
  3. cannot be detected in the peripheral blood
  4. enhances the production of glucagon

Directions Summarized				
A	B	C	D	E
1,2,3	1,3	2,4	4	All are
only	only	only	only	correct

458. The pathogenetic mechanism of acute pancreatitis caused by chronic alcoholism is most probably
    1. direct injury of pancreatic acini
    2. stimulation and activation of trypsinogen
    3. direct activation of proteolysis and lipolysis
    4. induction of partial pancreatic duct obstruction

459. Primary hyperaldosteronism characteristically manifest(s)
    1. hypokalemic alkalosis
    2. an adrenocortical adenoma
    3. hypertension
    4. increased levels of plasma renin

460. True statement(s) concerning hypopituitarism include(s)
    1. pituitary hypofunction is unlikely to occur until 75% of the gland is destroyed
    2. the temporal sequence of impairment of hormone production is the following: gonadotropins, growth hormone, TSH, ACTH, and prolactin
    3. Sheehan's pituitary necrosis is one of the most common causes of hypopituitarism
    4. lesions of the hypothalamus have been known to result in hypopituitarism

461. Multiple endocrine neoplasia (MEN) type I (Wermer's syndrome) is characterized by
    1. pituitary adenoma
    2. medullary carcinoma of the thyroid
    3. parathyroid adenoma
    4. pheochromocytoma of the adrenal

DIRECTIONS: Each set of lettered headings below is followed by a list of numbered words or phrases. For each numbered word or phrase select

- **A** if the item is associated with (A) *only*
- **B** if the item is associated with (B) *only*
- **C** if the item is associated with *both* (A) *and* (B)
- **D** if the item is associated with *neither* (A) *nor* (B)

Questions 462 – 467:

- **A.** Insulin-dependent diabetes mellitus (IDDM)
- **B.** Non-insulin-dependent diabetes mellitus (NIDDM)
- **C.** Both
- **D.** Neither

462. Significant reduction in the first and second phases of insulin response to a glucose load

463. HLA-D/DR antigens and autoimmune reaction

464. Normal or elevated absolute-fasting insulin level

465. A decrease in the number of insulin receptors in hepatocytes

466. Amyloidosis of islets of Langerhans

467. Necrotizing papillitis

Answers and Comments

448. C. Cyst formation may occur in any portion of the uninvoluted thyroglossal duct and it may be located anywhere from the base of the tongue to the suprasternal region in the midline. The lining is usually ciliated, pseudostratified columnar epithelium but it may undergo squamous metaplasia secondary to inflammation. (REF. 5, p. 1416)

449. E. Medullary carcinoma is derived from parafollicular or C cells of the thyroid. By electron microscopy the normal C cells (as well as the cells of medullary carcinoma) contain secretory granules of thyrocalcitonin. The elaboration of histaminase has become a useful test for the detection of medullary carcinoma, particularly when metastases are present. (REF. 5, pp. 1430–1433; REF. 1, pp. 1222–1223)

450. E. The histologic type most often encountered is the papillary type. More common in girls than boys by a ratio of 3:1, about 80% of these patients have a history of previous irradiation to the neck region for the treatment of a variety of benign conditions. The tumor may metastasize and cause death in some. (REF. 5, pp. 1427–1434)

451. C. Hyperprolactinemia is the most common endocrinopathy caused by pituitary tumors. The tumors are usually symptomatic early and, in women, present with amenorrhea-galactorrhea syndrome; however, local pressure effects usually bring affected men to medical attention. Treatment is by surgery, irradiation, or the administration of bromocriptine. (REF. 1, pp. 1194–1197)

452. D. Measurements of plasma blood glucose can be used to determine acute changes of the diabetic state. For long-term control, however, the measurement of glycosylated hemoglobin has proved more useful. Glucose can react nonenzymatically with several proteins including HbA, albumin, collagen, and lens crystallin. HbA_{1c}, which usually comprises about 3%–6% of total hemoglobin, increases severalfold in diabetes mellitus depending on the level of hyperglycemia. This measurement provides an index for blood glucose level for the previous 60–90 days. (REF. 3, p. 175)

453. C. Usually associated with acute pancreatitis, pancreatic pseudocysts may also arise following trauma to the abdomen. These cysts lack an epithelial lining and the wall is composed of fibrous tissue, which contains inflammatory cells. (REF. 1, p. 968)

454. D. The evidence for implicating autoimmunity in the pathogenesis of Graves' disease of the thyroid include the following: presence of microsomal autoantibodies in about 85% of patients, and the demonstration of thyroid-stimulating immunoglobulins and thyroid-growth immunoglobulins, probably responsible for hyperfunction of follicular cells and hyperplasia of the thyroid acini. (REF. 6, p. 681)

455. C. Antimicrosomal antibodies occur in about 95% of patients with Hashimoto's thyroiditis. In the pathogenesis of this disease, it is postulated that there is an organ-specific defect in suppressor T-cell function that enables the proliferation of a clone of B lymphocytes, which produce autoantibodies to the microsomal component of the thyroid cell, to thyroglobulin, and to the TSH receptors. (REF. 6, p. 679)

456. C. 21-hydroxylase deficiency is only minimal in the simple virilizing forms and severe in the salt-losing form of congenital hyperplasia of the adrenal cortex. In both forms there is overproduction of adrenal androgens which leads to macrogenitosomia precox in boys and pseudohermaphroditism in girls. (REF. 1, pp. 1241–1242)

457. A. A tetradecapeptide with a disulfide bond, somatostatin is a hormone derived from the D cells of the pancreatic islets. It is also found in the hypothalamus, gastric mucosa, and intestine. It inhibits the secretion of a variety of nonendocrine and endocrine substances including growth hormone, gastric acid, and insulin. Patients with D-cell tumors (somatostatinomas) present with hyperglycemia, malabsorption, and achlorhydria. (REF. 3, p. 167)

458. D. Chronic alcoholism or cholelithiasis induces duct obstruction and biliary/duodenal reflux into the pancreatic ducts.

Chronic alcoholism induces pancreatic obstruction through an increased protein concentration of pancreatic secretions with subsequent formation of inspissated plugs. (REF. 1, pp. 963–965)

459. D. Also known as Conn's syndrome, primary aldosteronism reveals sodium retention, expansion of the extracellular fluid compartment with subsequent suppression of renin production. In addition to adenoma, the adrenals may be hyperplastic or rarely show an adrenocortical carcinoma. (REF. 1, pp. 1240–1241)

460. E. Sheehan's syndrome is usually caused by postpartum hemorrhage and hypotension which precipitates the ischemic necrosis of the anterior pituitary. Other pathogenetic mechanisms that have been suggested include disseminated intravascular coagulation, sickle cell disease, vasculitis, and cavernous sinus thrombosis. (REF. 1, pp. 1196–1198)

461. B. Hyperplasia, adenoma, and/or carcinoma of the pituitary, parathyroid, and pancreatic islets constitute the chief characteristic features of MEN I (Wermer's syndrome), which is inherited as an autosomal dominant trait. Most of the lesions are functioning and patients present with a variety of clinical syndromes, among them Zollinger-Ellinson syndrome, parathyroidism, and prolactin-secreting pituitary tumor. MEN II (Sipple syndrome), on the other hand, comprises medullary carcinoma of the thyroid, pheochromocytoma with or without parathyroid hyperplasia. (REF. 6, p. 701; REF. 2, p. 1391)

462. B. In the patient with mild NIDDM, the response of the first phase of insulin response (0–10 min following a glucose challenge) is blunted and the second phase (10–12 min) is relatively normal. In those with severe disease, both phases are abnormal leading to significant hypoglycemia. (REF. 1, p. 979)

463. A. Evidence exists for pancreatic autoimmunity in IDDM. Antibodies against cytoplasmic and cell-membrane components of islet cells have been demonstrated. The presence of HLA-D/DR antigens in patients with IDDM may reflect the presence of HLA-lr genes which facilitate autoimmune responses. (REF. 1, p. 979)

464. B. Diabetic patients show abnormal response to the two phases of insulin response to the glucose challenge indicating an absolute deficiency of insulin. In spite of this the fasting insulin level is "normal even in patients with severe hypoglycemia. It could be said that the insulin level is relatively low for the needs of the abnormal levels of blood glucose. (REF. 1, p. 979)

465. B. Tissue resistance to the effects of insulin has been implicated in the pathogenesis of NIDDM. A decrease in the number of insulin receptors has also been described in monocytes, erythrocytes, and fat cells. (REF. 1, p. 980)

466. C. The amyloid deposit demonstrates the usual tintorial characteristics of this extracellular material. It should be distinguished from collagenous fibrosis. (REF. 1, p. 982)

467. C. The kidney is one of numerous organs that bear the brunt of diabetes mellitus. In addition to lesions of the small vessels and glomeruli, the kidneys may show bacterial infection in the form of pyelonephritis and necrotizing papillitis. (REF. 1, p. 984)

9 Skin and Breast

468. The most common predisposing factor for squamous cell carcinoma of the skin is
    A. stasis ulcers
    B. chronic sinuses of osteomyelitis
    C. prolonged contact with hydrocarbons
    D. chronic sun exposure in fair-complexioned individuals
    E. prolonged gamma radiation injury

469. Which of the following hormone receptor patterns of a breast tumor will show the highest response rates to endocrine ablation?
    A. Estrogen receptor-positive; progesterone receptor-negative
    B. Estrogen receptor-negative; progesterone receptor-positive
    C. Estrogen receptor-positive; progesterone receptor-positive
    D. Estrogen receptor-negative; progesterone receptor-negative
    E. None of the above

470. The most common type of infiltrating breast carcinoma is
    A. scirrhous
    B. medullary
    C. colloid
    D. Paget's disease
    E. lobular

471. With immunofluorescence techniques, the presence of antibodies against the basement membrane can be demonstrated in
    A. benign mucosal pemphigoid
    B. bullous pemphigoid
    C. pemphigus vulgaris
    D. pemphigus foliaceus
    E. localized chronic pemphigoid

472. In bullous pemphigoid, formation of bullae is observed in
    A. subcorneal location
    B. suprabasal location
    C. subepidermal location
    D. intradermal location
    E. within the stratum granulosum

473. Which of the following statements concerning lobular neoplasia of the breast (lobular carcinoma-in-situ) is NOT true?
    A. It generally presents as a mass
    B. It is frequently diagnosed incidentally in biopsies of breast taken for other reasons
    C. It generally shows multifocal origin
    D. The neoplastic epithelium is confined to mammary lobules and ducts
    E. It does not have a potential for distant metastases

474. In Clark's classification of levels of invasion of malignant melanomas, level III refers to the involvement by the neoplastic cells of
   A. superficial epidermis
   B. papillary dermis
   C. papillary-reticular dermal interface
   D. reticular dermis
   E. subcutaneous tissues

475. All of the histopathological findings of the following are similar EXCEPT
   A. herpes simplex
   B. varicella
   C. herpes zoster
   D. dermatitis herpetiformis
   E. variola

476. All of the viral inclusions of the following diseases are intranuclear EXCEPT
   A. herpes zoster
   B. verruca vulgaris
   C. molluscum contagiosum
   D. verruca plantaris
   E. verruca plana

477. The Munro microabscesses in psoriasis are located within the
   A. parakeratotic horny layer
   B. rete ridges
   C. upper dermis
   D. mid-dermis
   E. granular layer

478. A skin lesion characterized by acanthosis, prominent parakeratosis, thin epidermal plates over elongated papillae, absent or diminished stratum granulosum, Munro abscesses, and which reveals a positive Auspitz's sign is diagnostic of
   A. lichen planus
   B. actinic keratosis
   C. pemphigus vulgaris
   D. keratoacanthoma
   E. psoriasis

479. The most common type of skin cancer occurring after radiotherapy is
  - **A.** basal cell carcinoma
  - **B.** malignant melanoma
  - **C.** carcinoma of skin adnexae
  - **D.** squamous cell carcinoma
  - **E.** Kaposi's sarcoma

DIRECTIONS: For each of the questions or incomplete statements below, **one** or **more** of the answers or completions given is correct. Select
  - **A** if only *1, 2, and 3* are correct
  - **B** if only *1 and 3* are correct
  - **C** if only *2 and 4* are correct
  - **D** if only *4* is correct
  - **E** if all are correct

---

480. The Tzanck test is of value in diagnosing
  1. herpes simplex
  2. impetigo
  3. varicella
  4. dermatitis herpetiformis

481. Which of the following is (are) true statement(s) regarding Paget's disease of the breast?
  1. Intraductal carcinoma invariably antedates the skin changes
  2. Invasion of the dermal lymphatics by malignant cells is its histologic hallmark
  3. Eczematoid changes occur in the nipple and areola
  4. It is referred to clinically as inflammatory carcinoma

482. Gynecomastia may be one of the manifestations of
  1. cirrhosis of the liver
  2. Klinefelter's syndrome
  3. starvation
  4. Turner's syndrome

483. Which of the following is (are) characteristic feature(s) of carcinoma arising in the male breast?
   1. Rapid infiltration of the underlying thoracic wall
   2. Axillary lymph node involvement in approximately one-half of the cases at the time of presentation
   3. Ulceration through the skin is more common than in the female
   4. Less scirrhous quality of the tumor than in female breast cancer

484. Erythema nodosum may be a manifestation of
   1. syphilis
   2. leprosy
   3. coccidioidomycosis
   4. cat-scratch fever

485. Which of the following statements concerning basal cell carcinoma is (are) true?
   1. If untreated, this neoplasm will erode and infiltrate the neighboring tissues, including cartilage and bone
   2. The tip of the nose is the most frequent site
   3. A tendency towards desmoplasia is seen in tumors located away from the face
   4. It behaves more aggressively if located above the anal verge of the anal canal

---

DIRECTIONS: Each group of questions below consists of five lettered headings followed by a list of numbered words, phrases, or statements. For **each** numbered word, phrase, or statement, select the **one** lettered heading that is most closely associated with it. Each lettered heading may be selected once, more than once, or not at all.

Questions 486 – 490:
   A. Acanthosis
   B. Parakeratosis
   C. Acantholysis
   D. Hyperkeratosis
   E. Pseudoepitheliomatous hyperplasia

486. Loss of cohesion of keratinocytes resulting from destruction of desmosomes

487. Thickened epidermis secondary to proliferation of the prickle cell layer

488. Exaggerated reactive epidermal hyperplasia, with disorganized pattern at the dermoepidermal junction

489. Thickened stratum corneum associated with prominent granular layer

490. Retention of nuclei in cells of stratum corneum associated with diminished or absent granular layer

Questions 491 – 496:
  A. Medullary carcinoma
  B. Inflammatory carcinoma
  C. Cystosarcoma phyllodes
  D. Scirrhous carcinoma
  E. Tubular carcinoma

491. Infiltration of subepidermal lymphatics and vessels by tumor

492. Diffuse brawny induration; usually no definable tumor mass

493. Desmoplastic stromal reaction

494. Metastases to lungs rather than to axillary nodes

495. Benign epithelial clefts; malignant stroma

496. Dense hyalinized stroma diffusely infiltrated by small clusters, small glands, and ribbons or single rows of cancer cells

Answers and Comments

468. D. Among the varied predisposing factors mentioned in question 468, chronic sun exposure in fair-complexioned persons is most common. When squamous cell carcinoma occurs on sun-exposed skin signs of actinic keratosis (solar keratosis), a premalignant lesion, are almost always present in the adjacent skin. (REF. 1, p. 1266)

469. C. The presence or absence of cytoplasmic estrogen and progesterone receptors in breast tumors is used to predict and monitor the response of metastatic breast carcinoma to procedures which reduce the levels of such hormones. The highest response rates to endocrine ablation are observed in patients with tumors containing both receptors. (REF. 1, p. 1188)

470. A. Over 90% of breast carcinomas arise within the ducts. Scirrhous, medullary, colloid, and Paget's disease are major variants of infiltrating duct carcinoma. In approximately 75% of the invasive duct carcinomas there are no distinguishing histologic features except for the increased fibrous tissue stroma giving the tumor a hard consistency on gross examination (thus the term scirrhous carcinoma). Because some invasive lobular carcinomas have scirrhous gross features it was suggested that the more common infiltrating scirrhous duct carcinoma be referred to as infiltrating duct carcinoma, simple or usual type. The incidence of infiltrating lobular carcinoma is 4.9%. (REF. 1, p. 1181)

471. B. With immunofluorescence studies performed on frozen biopsy specimens, the localization of IgE in the dermoepidermal basement membrane zone has been demonstrated. In pemphigus vulgaris, the localization of IgE is observed in the region of epithelial intercellular cement substance and is absent in the dermo-epidermal basement membrane zone. (REF. 1, pp. 1294–1295)

472. C. The earliest changes in bullous pemphigoid are observed in the apical zones of dermal papillae; the formation of microvacuoles beneath the basal layer is followed by dermo-epidermal dehiscence and formation of bullae. The rete ridges frequently show effacement. The dermo-epidermal separation leads to outpouring of plasma-containing fibrin and inflammatory cells in the newly formed bullae. (REF. 1, p. 1295)

473. A. Lobular neoplasia (lobular carcinoma-in-situ) of the breast is a histological entity; however, more recently mammography is proving to become an important diagnostic modality. Since the lesion does not produce a palpable mass, it is diagnosed incidentally during examination of breast sections for other benign or malignant lesions. (REF. 2, p. 1555)

474. C. Clark's classification of levels of invasion of malignant melanoma has gained widespread acceptance in recent years. An important correlation between the prognosis and the depth of invasion of these lesions has been shown. Clark's classification can be summarized as follows:

Level I, intraepithelial melanoma; level II, invasion of papillary dermis by melanoma cells; level III, the tumor grows along the papillary-reticular dermis interface and its cells appear to impinge upon, but do not break through, the collagen bundles of the reticular dermis; level IV, involvement of reticular dermis; level V, involvement of subcutaneous tissue. (REF. 5, pp. 191–192)

475. D. Dermatitis herpetiformis, which is of unknown etiology, produces a subepidermal bulla owing to basal cell degeneration. Psychogenic factors are felt to play a role in this disease, and most patients respond to the administration of sulfapyridine. The other diseases are of viral origin and, aside from the characteristic viral inclusion bodies, produce ballooning degeneration resulting in acantholysis and intraepidermal bullae. (REF. 1, pp. 1293–1297)

476. C. The large (up to 35 μm) homogeneous, eosinophilic intracytoplasmic inclusion in molluscum contagiosum contain replicating virions. (REF. 1, pp. 1298–1299)

477. A. The Munro abscesses located within parakerototic areas of horny layer represent accumulation of neutrophils that have migrated from capillaries in the papilla through the suprapapillary epidermis. (REF. 1, p. 1292)

478. E. In addition to the features enumerated, psoriasis shows elongated clubbed rete ridges, rigid vessels in the dermal papillae, and dermal infiltration with lymphocytes and histiocytes. The clinical distribution and presentation of the lesions form the basis for the classification of psoriasis into P. guttata, P. rupoides, P. follicularis, and P. nummularis. (REF. 2, pp. 1589–1590)

479. D. Although basal cell carcinomas may occur after radiotherapy, squamous carcinomas are the most frequent type. Spindle cell carcinomas are an anaplastic variety of squamous cell carcinomas produced by irradiation. (REF. 1, p. 467)

480. B. The Tzanck test may be useful in making a rapid preliminary diagnosis. The presence of multinucleated giant cells in herpes simplex, herpes zoster, varicella, and pemphigus is pathognomonic of these bullous diseases. (REF. 1, p. 284)

481. B. Paget's disease of the breast is a form of duct carcinoma that arises in the main excretory ducts of the breast and subsequently invades the skin of the nipple and areola. The malignant invasion of the skin of the nipple and areola results in characteristic gross features such as hyperemia, edema, development of fissures, ulceration, and oozing (eczematoid changes). Inflammatory carcinoma is a special tumor only by virtue of its clinical findings which closely resemble an acute inflammation of the breast; its histologic characteristics are not specific but invasion of the subepidermal lymphatics and vessels is the identifying feature. (REF. 1, pp. 1181–1184)

482. A. Enlargement of the male breast (gynecomastia) is usually caused by hormonal imbalance, with absolute or relative increase in estrogenic hormones. When occurring in old age, with cirrhosis of the liver, starvation, and in hypogonadal syndromes (i.e., Klinefelter), gynecomastia is related to a decrease in the testosterone:estradiol ratio. Individuals with Turner's syndrome are phenotypically female but fail to develop normal secondary sex characteristics at puberty due to atrophic fibrous ovaries (streaks). (REF. 1, p. 1189)

483. E. Carcinoma of the male breast is very rare with a frequency ratio to breast cancer in the female of 1:100. Rapid infiltration of the underlying thoracic wall and overlying skin occurs because of the scant amount of breast substance in the male. Breast cancer in the male has less striking desmoplasia than in the female but follows the same pattern of dissemination as in women. (REF. 1, p. 1189)

484. E. The tender, pale-red to purplish-blue nodules of erythema nodosum are commonly located on the anterior aspect of the lower extremities. This disease is a manifestation of a variety of unrelated infections that also include measles and ringworm. It may follow lymphomas, administration of vaccine, and the ingestion of drugs. (REF. 1, pp. 1288–1289)

485. B. Basal cell carcinomas occur predominantly on the face, bounded by the upper lip, ears, and hairline, in blond, fair-skinned people. Tumors at the tip of the nose are more likely to be squamous carcinomas. Squamous cell carcinomas of the anal canal may appear histologically similar to basal cell carcinomas. (REF. 1, pp. 1265–1266)

486. C. The epidermal cells are attached to each other by focal specializations of their walls called desmosomes. Destruction of the desmosomes, thus the attachments, causes the cells to lose their cohesiveness. This process is termed acantholysis. (REF. 1, p. 1261)

487. A. Pseudoepitheliomatous hyperplasia is an excessive form of acanthosis, producing a disorganized pattern at the dermoepidermal junction. (REF. 1, p. 1261)

488. E. See explanatory answer 487. (REF 2, p. 1576)

489. D. Parakeratosis and hyperkeratosis are manifestations of abnormal keratinization; parakeratosis represents incomplete keratinization. (REF. 2, p. 1575)

490. B. See explanatory answer 489. (REF. 2, p. 1576)

491. B. Inflammatory carcinoma earned its name through its characteristically close resemblance to acute mastitis. More than three fourths of the patients have axillary metastases at the time of consultation. (REF. 2, p. 1566)

492. B. See explanatory answer 491. (REF. 2, p. 1566)

493. D. So named because of its hard and gritty gross characteristics, scirrhous carcinoma is identified histologically by a dense hyalinized stroma diffusely infiltrated by columns or nests of malignant cells. The hardness is primarily due to desmoplastic stromal response. (REF. 2, p. 1561)

494. C. A malignant counterpart of fibroadenoma, cystosarcoma phyllodes consists of long narrow slits of benign epithelial channels and a benign cellular or sarcomatous stroma. The latter may be a liposarcoma, fibrosarcoma, osteosarcoma, leiomyosarcoma, or a combination of sarcomas. Vascular route of dissemination is the rule, and pulmonary metastases are frequent sequelae. (REF. 2, pp. 1550–1551)

495. C. See explanatory answer 494. (REF. 2, p. 1551)

496. D. See explanatory answer 493. (REF. 2, p. 1561)

10 Central Nervous and Musculoskeletal Systems

DIRECTIONS: Each of the questions or incomplete statements below is followed by five suggested answers or completions. Select the **one** that is best in each case.

497. A fatal outcome in poliomyelitis is usually attributable to
    A. necrotizing encephalitis
    B. marked increase in intracranial pressure
    C. involvement of the nervous system mechanisms controlling respiration
    D. severe myocarditis
    E. swelling, fragmentation, and destruction of axons in white matter

498. Which of the following brain infections is LEAST likely to leave behind residual damage?
    A. Congenital toxoplasmosis
    B. Encephalitis lethargica
    C. St. Louis encephalitis
    D. Eastern equine encephalitis
    E. Herpes simplex

499. Which of the following is diagnostic of rabies?
    A. Enlarged microglia containing inclusions
    B. Widespread neuronal loss with "windswept" cortex
    C. Petechial hemorrhages in limbic region
    D. Intracytoplasmic eosinophilic round or bullet-shaped inclusions in nerve cells
    E. Loss of Purkinje's cells

500. The incubation period of rabies is variable and seems to be related to
    A. the infecting dose of the virus
    B. the type of vector
    C. vaccination
    D. the distance between wound and the brain or spinal cord
    E. clinical disease in the vector

501. Lymphocytic choriomeningitis is
    A. characterized by intense lymphocytic infiltration, which is limited to the leptomeninges
    B. usually fatal in man
    C. diagnosed only when the virus is isolated
    D. characterized by moderate lymphocytic infiltrate limited to the subependymal vessels
    E. probably transmitted to man through the urine of infected mice

502. Which of the following is histologically indistinguishable from seminoma?
    A. Medulloblastoma
    B. Astrocytoma, grade I
    C. Oligodenodroglioma
    D. Pineal germinoma
    E. Astrocytoma, grade II

503. In children, medulloblastomas usually originate in the region of
   A. cerebellar vermis
   B. cerebral hemispheres
   C. fourth ventricle
   D. pons
   E. filum terminale

504. All of the following are characteristic histological features of glioblastoma multiforme EXCEPT
   A. profuse numbers of large pleomorphic and often bizarre cells with abundant abnormal mitoses
   B. large and small areas of necrosis, usually with garlands of small nuclei at the periphery
   C. vascular proliferation with endothelial and adventitial hyperplasia
   D. diffuse proliferation of polygonal cells without a characteristic pattern, except for few cells whose processes radiate around blood vessels
   E. some areas with small cells resembling oat cell carcinoma of lung

505. In patients younger than 60 years paralysis agitans is characterized by generalized brain atrophy and
   A. neurofibrillary tangles
   B. Lewy bodies
   C. disseminated focal astrocytic scars
   D. loss of large cells of the caudate nuclei
   E. loss of large cells of the putamen

506. In Wilson's disease, free copper is deposited in the
   A. corpus striatum
   B. globus pallidus
   C. inferior olivary nucleus
   D. dentate nucleus
   E. hippocampus

507. Which of the following is NOT true of fibrous dysplasia of the bone?
  A. Usual occurrence in metaphysis
  B. Most commonly affects the humerus
  C. Association in polyostotic type with precocious puberty in females
  D. Abnormal morphology of bone spicules
  E. Usual appearance in late childhood

508. All of the following are well-known causes of generalized osteoporosis EXCEPT
  A. hyperparathyroidism
  B. rheumatoid arthritis
  C. hyperthyroidism
  D. hyperadrenocorticism
  E. acromegaly

509. The initial and basic pathologic change in osteoarthritis (degenerative joint disease) is
  A. degeneration of articular cartilage
  B. chronic inflammation of the synovium
  C. reduction in the volume of synovial fluid
  D. degenerative changes in the subchondral bone
  E. acute inflammation of the synovium

510. The mechanism of hydrocephalus caused by the Arnold-Chiari malformation is
  A. inflammatory
  B. overproduction of cerebrospinal fluid
  C. deficient resorption of cerebrospinal fluid
  D. obstructive
  E. unknown

511. The commonest cause of acute leptomeningitis in infants and children is
  A. *Hemophilus influenzae*
  B. *Neisseria meningitidis*
  C. *Staphylococcus aureus*
  D. *Streptococcus pneumoniae*
  E. *Streptococcus viridans*

512. Which of the following is most unlikely to cause intracerebral hemorrhage?
   A. Blood dyscrasias
   B. Atherosclerosis
   C. Berry aneurysms
   D. Hypertensive vascular disease
   E. Trauma

513. Arterial bleeding is the usual cause of
   A. acute subdural hematoma
   B. chronic subdural hematoma
   C. epidural hematoma
   D. subarachnoid hematoma
   E. subdural hygroma

514. Diagnostic rosettes composed of tumor cells arranged in a ring around a space to create a tubule are found in
   A. glioblastoma multiforme
   B. ependymoma
   C. oligodendroglioma
   D. low-grade astrocytoma
   E. fibroblastic meningioma

515. Which of the following diseases is not characterized primarily by demyelination?
   A. Multiple sclerosis
   B. Neuromyelitis optica (Devic's disease)
   C. Postinfectious encephalitis
   D. Progressive multifocal leukoencephalopathy
   E. Alzheimer's disease

516. All of these are characteristic of Wallerian degeneration EXCEPT
   A. results from ischemic injury to the neuron
   B. the cell body undergoes chromatolysis
   C. there is distal degeneration of the axon
   D. degeneration of the myelin sheath may occur
   E. may show regeneration of nerve sprouts

DIRECTIONS: For each of the questions or incomplete statements below, **one** or **more** of the answers or completions given is correct. Select

    A if only *1, 2, and 3* are correct
    B if only *1 and 3* are correct
    C if only *2 and 4* are correct
    D if only *4* is correct
    E if all are correct

---

517. Intranuclear inclusions may be found in the encephalitis caused by
    1. measles virus
    2. herpes simplex virus
    3. cytomegalic inclusion virus
    4. herpes zoster virus

518. In the primary response of the brain parenchyma to injury, reactive changes are seen involving which of the following?
    1. Microglia
    2. Oligodendrocytes
    3. Astrocytes
    4. Fibrocytes

519. The lesions of Parkinson's disease are confined to
    1. substantia nigra
    2. locus ceruleus
    3. dorsal nucleus of the vagus
    4. subcortical gray areas of the cerebellum

520. Large cerebral infarcts may be associated with
    1. atherosclerosis with thrombosis
    2. atherosclerosis without thrombosis
    3. emboli in large arteries
    4. venous occlusion

521. Cerebral hemorrhage secondary to uncontrolled hypertension primarily affects the
 1. lenticular nucleus
 2. thalamus
 3. internal capsule
 4. medulla

522. Common extra-articular manifestation(s) of rheumatoid arthritis is (are)
 1. rheumatoid nodules
 2. pannus formation
 3. tenosynovitis
 4. rheumatoid geodes

523. Which of the following renal change(s) may be seen in gout?
 1. Formation of tophi within the pyramids
 2. Tubular precipitates of uric acid
 3. Nephrosclerosis
 4. Pyelonephritis

524. Muscle atrophy occurs in
 1. immobilization of an extremity
 2. thiamine chloride deficiency
 3. Buerger's disease
 4. hyperaldosteronism

525. Muscular dystrophies characterized by proximal limb weakness and autosomal dominant inheritance are
 1. fascioscapulo humeral dystrophy
 2. Duchenne dystrophy
 3. scapuloperoneal dystrophy
 4. Becker dystrophy

526. Osteoid osteoma is characterized by
 1. disproportionate degree of pain compared to its size
 2. involvement predominantly of flat bones
 3. extremely rare incidence in patients over 40 years
 4. x-ray pattern of sclerotic "nidus"

Directions Summarized

A	B	C	D	E
1,2,3	1,3	2,4	4	All are
only	only	only	only	correct

527. Chondrocalcinosis articularis is characterized by
    1. deposition of urate crystals
    2. deposition of calcium pyrophosphate dihydrate crystals
    3. deposition of xanthine crystals
    4. recurrent synovitis primarily involving large joints

528. Osteosarcoma can occur in
    1. previously normal bone
    2. Paget's disease of the bone
    3. hereditary multiple exostosis
    4. previously irradiated bone

529. Which of the following histologic feature(s) is (are) seen in cases of dystrophic calcification?
    1. Calcium salts have a basophilic, amorphous, granular, and sometimes clumped appearance in the usual tissue stain
    2. Heterotopic bone may be formed in the focus of calcification
    3. Occasionally single necrotic cells may constitute seed crystals that become encrusted by the mineral deposits
    4. Psammoma bodies may be present

530. Dystrophic calcification is frequently encountered in
    1. chronic tuberculosis
    2. centers of large infarcts
    3. aging atheromas of advanced atherosclerosis
    4. hyperparathyroidism

531. Osteoporosis is characterized by
    1. normal serum calcium
    2. impaired mineralization of bone
    3. involvement of the entire skeleton
    4. elevated alkaline phosphatase

532. The following is (are) true of Lyme disease.
1. It is believed that the disease is immunologically derived
2. Cardiac and neurological abnormalities may develop
3. Involvement of the joints is a cardinal sign in over half of the patients
4. The disease is caused by an adenovirus

533. In myaesthenia gravis,
1. thymomas outnumber thymic hyperplasia 2:1 in affected patients
2. antibodies to acetylcholine receptors are produced at the neuromuscular junction
3. muscle biopsy characteristically shows severe muscle atrophy
4. IgG and C3 are demonstrable at the myoneural junction by immunoperoxidase technique

534. Involvement of the dorsal root ganglion is characteristic for
1. rabies
2. herpes simplex
3. poliomyelitis
4. herpes zoster

535. Multiple sclerosis is characterized by
1. demyelination
2. loss of oligodendroglia
3. perivascular aggregation of lymphocytes and histiocytes
4. pronounced astrocytosis

536. Which of the following may be encountered in Landry-Guillain-Barre syndrome?
1. Acute demyelination
2. Combined motor and sensory neuropathy
3. An elevated CSF protein associated with a normal cell count
4. Involvement of the temporal lobes

Directions Summarized				
A	B	C	D	E
1,2,3	1,3	2,4	4	All are
only	only	only	only	correct

537. Patients with which of the following are at risk for osteogenic sarcoma?
  1. Paget's disease of bone
  2. Multiple enchondromatosis
  3. Hereditary retinoblastoma
  4. Fibrous dysplasia of bone

DIRECTIONS: The group of questions below consists of five lettered headings followed by a list of numbered words, phrases, or statements. For **each** numbered word, phrase, or statement, select the **one** lettered heading that is most closely associated with it. Each lettered heading may be selected once, more than once, or not at all.

Questions 538–542:
  A. Ostecmalacia
  B. Osteopetrosis
  C. Ollier's disease
  D. Paget's disease
  E. Osgood-Schlatter disease

538. Anemia, hepatosplenomegaly, "brittle" bones

539. Aseptic necrosis of tibial tubercle

540. Enchondromatosis

541. Inadequate mineralization of bone matrix; decreased appositional growth rate

542. Excessive bone resorption, deposition of irregular woven bone, replacement of marrow by loose vascularized fibrous tissue

Questions 543–549:
- **A.** Intracranial neurilemmoma
- **B.** Colloid cyst
- **C.** Craniopharyngioma
- **D.** Sturge-Weber-Dimitri disease
- **E.** Déjerine-Sottas disease

543. Persistence of embryonic paraphyseal pouch

544. Limited to roof of third ventricle

545. Vestibular portion of eighth nerve

546. Schwann cells

547. Erdheim cell rests

548. Mineralization of cortical vessels gives characteristic x-ray pattern

549. Onion skin-like layering of connective tissue around peripheral axon

Questions 550–555:
- **A.** Creutzfeldt-Jacob disease
- **B.** Alzheimer's disease
- **C.** Brain abscess
- **D.** Intracerebral hemorrhage
- **E.** Subarachnoid hemorrhage

550. Cyanotic congenital heart disease

551. "Bubbles and holes" in the cerebral cortex, associated with progressive severe dementia with myoclonus

552. Berry aneurysm

553. Cortical atrophy, hydrocephalus ex vacuo associated with severe dementia

554. Hypertension

555. Microaneurysms of Charcot-Bouchard

Answers and Comments

497. C. Death in poliomyelitis is generally due to a respiratory failure. The lesions responsible for this may be central, affecting the respiratory center in the medulla, or peripheral, involving the anterior horn cells supplying the intercostal and the diaphragmatic musculature. (REF. 1, p. 1385)

498. C. The prognosis of St. Louis encephalitis generally is excellent. Complete recovery without any residual sequelae is commonly seen. Residual damage is frequently seen following recovery from toxoplasmosis, encephalitis lethargica, and Eastern equine encephalitis. (REF. 1, p. 1383)

499. D. The pathognomonic Negri bodies are the intraneuronal, intracytoplasmic, eosinophilic inclusion bodies, which may vary in their configuration from round to oval to bullet-shaped. Widespread neuronal loss with so-called windswept cortex is seen in neurosyphilis. (REF. 1, p. 1384)

500. D. It has been observed that the closer the distance of the wound (the portal of entry of the virus into the body) to the spinal cord and the brain, the shorter the incubation period. It seems probable that the virus travels along the neural pathways from the wound to the central nervous system. (REF. 1, p. 1384)

501. E. Lymphocytic choriomeningitis is rarely fatal in man, hence, the designation "benign lymphocytic meningitis." Infected mice act as host reservoirs. Moderate lymphocytic infiltrations on the leptomeninges, subependymal vessels, and choroid plexuses are characteristic features. Diagnosis is usually made by the presence of a rising titer of specific neutralizing antibodies. (REF. 2, pp. 355, 1910)

502. D. The germinoma of the pineal gland, pinealoma consists of two cell types: The large, pale polyhedral to spherical cells admixed with small nests of lymphocytelike cells. The cell types and their separation into lobules by vascular connective tissue trabeculae are identical to those seen in seminoma. (REF. 1, p. 1253)

503. A. A highly malignant and uniformly malignant neoplasm, medulloblastoma (neuroblastoma, granuloblastoma) represents 8% of all neuroglial neoplasms. It occurs predominantly in children; the greatest incidence is in those 5–9 years of age. Most of the tumors originate at the region of the cerebellar vermis, possibly from microscopic remnants of the cerebellar external granular layer. (REF. 1, pp. 1406–1407)

504. D. This describes a pattern seen in ependymoma. (REF. 1, pp. 1402–1403)

505. B. Parkinsonism is currently viewed as a symptom complex most frequently of viral or idiopathic etiology. The term paralysis agitans is usually reserved for the idiopathic variety and is characterized by generalized brain atrophy and the presence of single or multiple round, hyaline, eosinophilic intracytoplasmic inclusions (Lewy bodies). Neurofibrillary tangles and astrocytic scars are more suggestive of the inflammatory type. Such distinctions are easier in lesions of younger people as compared to older individuals. D and E have been described in patients with either type of Parkinsonism but are not generally accepted as diagnostic features. (REF. 2, p. 1895)

506. A. As a result of the absence or deficiency of serum alpha-globulin ceruloplasmin, the bound and total serum copper is low and the free copper is deposited in the liver (micronodular cirrhosis), Descemet's membrane of the eye (Kayser-Fleischer rings), putamen, and striate bodies. The last two sites are the areas discolored by bile pigments in kernicterus. (REF. 1, p. 1423)

507. B. Fibrous dysplasia, a nonneoplastic bone disorder, is divided into the more common monostotic type and the usual variant, the polyostotic type. The polyostotic variety is usually associated with endocrine dysfunction, precocious puberty in females, and areas of hyperpigmentation of the skin. The monostotic type occurs frequently in older children and young adults and frequently affects the rib, femur, and tibia. Microscopically, narrow, curved, misshapened bone trabeculae ("fishhook" shape) are interspersed with fibrous tissue. (REF. 1, pp. 1333–1334; REF. 2, p. 1779)

508. B. Joint disease is the hallmark of rheumatoid arthritis; diffuse proliferative synovitis is the characteristic morphologic change. (REF. 1, pp. 1326–1329)

509. A. Unlike rheumatoid arthritis which is principally a disease of the synovium, osteoarthritis begins with degeneration of articular cartilage. Degradation of the matrix of the cartilage affecting chondroitin sulphate and other proteoglycans constitutes the mechanism of this change. Aging plays a dominant role in the pathogenesis; the possibility of immunologically mediated tissue injury combined with genetic factors have also been speculated upon. (REF. 6, pp. 715–716)

510. D. The Arnold-Chiari malformation consists of caudal displacement of the medulla and vermis of the cerebellum into the spinal canal below the level of the foramen magnum. It is usually associated with platybasia, a flattening of the base of the skull, and with meningomyelocele. Two major types of hydrocephalus are recognized: communicating and noncommunicating (obstructive). (REF. 1, p. 1377; REF. 2, pp. 1874–1875)

511. A. In hemophilus meningitis, similar to other acute bacterial leptomeningitis, the cerebrospinal fluid shows elevated pressure, decreased glucose, elevated protein, and exceedingly high neutrophilic count. The exudate, which may be found on the convex surface of the brain, is more prominent at the base of the brain. The most frequently encountered organism in the meningitis of neonates and young adults are *Escherischia coli* and *Neisseria meningitidis* respectively. (REF. 1, pp. 1378–1379)

512. B. The most common cause of intracerebral hemorrhage is hypertension occurring 10 to 20 times more frequently than other causes. The precise mechanism by which hypertension causes cerebrovascular accident is not known. Precipitation of the hemorrhage by rupture of small vessels or microaneurysms has been postulated. (REF. 1, p. 1392)

513. C. Because it results from arterial bleeding, epidural hematoma accumulates fast and causes rapidly progressive neurological symptoms and signs, usually within minutes or hours of trauma. Thus, it should be considered a surgical emergency.

Subdural hematomas result most frequently from a tear of the bridging veins between the dura and the cerebral cortex. Subdural hygroma is a collection of blood tinged CSF, usually a product of previous trauma. (REF. 1, pp. 1396–1398)

514. B. Also observed in ependymomas are pseudorosettes composed of tumor cells arranged around blood vessels. Most ependymomas are histologically benign and slow growing; their location, however, makes them inaccessible for surgical removal. (REF. 1, p. 1404)

515. E. Alzheimer's disease is a degenerative disease which typically shows progressive atrophy of the brain, particularly the frontal, parietal, and occipital cortices. Neurofibrillary tangles, senile plaques, and granulovacuolar degeneration of neurons are some of the microscopic alterations that may be seen in affected brains. (REF. 1, p. 1410)

516. A. Severance of an axon is followed by central chromatolysis and swelling of the cell body. The distal part of the severed axon undergoes dissolution with conversion of the myelin into fatty globules (Wallerian degeneration). Peripheral nerves may also be affected by two other distinct pathologic processes: axonal degeneration and segmental demyclination. (REF. 1, p. 1428)

517. E. Cowdry type A intranuclear inclusions may be found in affected nerve cells and glia in measles encephalitis; it may, more likely, be found in oligodendrocytes than in the rapidly destroyed neurons of herpesvirus encephalitis. In cytomegalic inclusions disease, the Cowdry type A intranuclear inclusions are large and prominent. (REF. 2, p. 1908)

518. A. Astrocytes, microglia, and oligodendrocytes are included in the category of glial cells. Glial cells serve the supportive and reparative functions in brain parenchyma. Fibrocytes may be involved in the reparative processes but only in the later stages. The fibrocytes are derived from the blood vessels and the meninges. (REF. 1, pp. 1373–1374)

519. A. The loss of pigment, characteristic of this disease, can be seen grossly and is the result of cellular destruction with phagocytosis and removal of the cell products and specific pigment. (REF. 2, p. 1895)

520. E. Dissecting hematoma, although rarely, may produce large infarctions through luminal compression of the affected artery. (REF. 1, pp. 1388–1391)

521. A. Approximately 70% of hemorrhages in hypertensive patients are in the medial or lateral ganglionic regions (lenticular nuclei, thalami, internal capsules). From these areas blood may flow along the nerve tracts to midbrain, pons, or into adjacent parietal and frontal lobes. About 20% occur in midbrain, pons, or white matter of the cerebellum. About 10% begin initially in the remaining portions of the cerebral hemispheres. The medulla is never the initial site of this type of hemorrhage and is only rarely involved by extension. (REF. 1, p. 1392)

522. B. Rheumatoid nodules are seen in approximately 20% of the patients and occur most often in tendons, tendon sheaths, and periarticular subcutaneous tissue. It can also be seen in the heart, large vessels, lung, pleura, kidney, meninges, and the synovial membrane itself. (REF. 1, p. 1352)

523. E. In recent studies, tubular damage followed by an interstitial reaction is the earliest structural abnormality in the kidney, thus, the morphological lesion that had been interpreted as pyelonephritis may not be of infectious origin. (REF. 1, pp. 1356–1361)

524. A. Hyperaldosteronism is associated with distinctive intracellular alterations such as hydropic vacuoles within the cells. (REF. 1, p. 1306)

525. B. Duchenne and Becker dystrophies are X-linked recessive diseases. (REF. 1, pp. 1308–1310)

526. B. The extreme pain of the small tumor is promptly relieved upon tumor removal. The x-ray pattern of osteolytic "nidus" enclosed within densely sclerotic reactive bone in a femur or tibia of an older child or adolescent is virtually diagnostic. (REF. 2, p. 1785)

527. C. The incidence of this disorder among males and females is approximately equal. Hyperuricemia and deposition of uric acid crystals are very rarely associated with this disorder. (REF. 1, p. 1362)

528. E. This tumor usually arises in preexisting normal bone. Fifteen percent arises in previously diseased bones, such as Paget's disease (6% of all osteosarcomas), previous irradiation (4% of all osteosarcomas), polyostotic fibrous dysplasia, enchondromas, and exostosis. (REF. 1, pp. 1337–1340)

529. E. Bodies formed by progressive acquisition of outer layers by which a laminated configuration is produced are called psammoma bodies because of their resemblance to grains of sand. Not infrequently, for reasons that are not clear, the calcification may produce bone formation, and at times this heterotopic bone may show islands of active marrow. (REF. 1, p. 35)

530. A. This alteration is principally encountered in areas of coagulation, caseous, enzymatic, and liquifactive necrosis, particularly when the necrotic tissue persists for long periods of time. The hypercalcemia of hyperparathyroidism may cause calcification in the normal tissue (metastatic calcification). (REF. 1, p. 35)

531. B. Predominantly a disease of postmenopausal women, but also occurring in men between the ages of 50 and 70 years, osteoporosis is characterized by an absolute reduction in the amount of bone necessary for mechanical support. The etiology is multifactorial, thus, the disease is classified as primary, when the etiology is not known and secondary in cases where there is association with a definite disease entity. In recent times the role of estrogen in the pathogenesis of osteoporosis has received much attention. (REF. 6, pp. 704–706)

532. A. Lyme disease (previously called Lyme arthritis) is a tick-borne multisystem disease caused by the spirochete, Borrelia burgdorferi. Three stages of evolution of the disease are identified: (1) dermatologic, with constitutional symptoms; (2) cardiac (AV block, pericarditis) and neurologic (meningitis, encephalitis), occurring in about 15% of patients; and (3) arthritis. It is thought to be an immune complex disease, immune complexes being demonstrable in involved joints. (REF. 6, pp. 714–715)

533. C. There are remarkably scanty alterations in the skeletal muscles in myaesthenia gravis (MG). Occasional myofiber atrophy or necrosis and scattered focal collections of lymphocytes may be observed. Autoantibodies to acetylcholine receptors are found in 85% of patients; these antibodies and C3 are demonstrable at the postsynaptic membrane of the neuromuscular junction. Thymic abnormalities are present in 70%–80% of patients: thymic hyperplasia in about 65% and thymoma in the remainder. (REF. 1, pp. 1310–1312)

534. D. Some viruses have a proclivity for infecting specific organs, tissues, or parts of the nervous system. Thus, poliomyelitis affects the anterior horn motor cells predominantly; herpes simplex has a predilection for neurons of the temporal lobe; and the virus of progressive multifocal leukoencephalopathy primarily infects oligodendrocytes. (REF. 1, p. 1382)

535. E. The gross pathologic hallmark of multiple sclerosis (MS) is the plaque, which typically is a well-delineated irregular lesion, which is found in the white and gray matter in the central nervous system. They may be faintly visible (shallow plaques), vary in color depending on the age of the plaque, and may vary from minute to large lesions. In addition to the microscopic features of MS enumerated in the questions, lipid-laden macrophages are observed; the axons within the involved areas are usually normal. (REF. 1, pp. 1410–1411)

536. A. Acute idiopathic polyneuritis (Guillain-Barre syndrome) is a disease of peripheral nerves characterized by acute demyelination, a history of "viral" prodrome in about 40% of affected patients, and a rapidly progressive motor neuropathy with variable sensory disturbances. The lesions, which are focal, contain lymphocytes and histiocytes. (REF. 1, pp. 1429–1430)

537. A. Most common between the ages of 10 and 25 years and affecting males twice as often as females, osteogenic sarcoma occurs frequently at the ends of long bones, particularly around the knee and the upper end of the humerus. Fibrous dysplasia, in which there is focal replacement of bone by fibrous tissue, may be associated with cafe-au-lait spots of the skin, a constellation of features known as Albright's syndrome. Malignant transformation of the lesion is rare. (REF. 6, pp. 708–710)

538. B. Osteopetrosis (osteosclerosis) is characterized by overgrowth and sclerosis of bone resulting in marked thickening of the bony cortex and narrowing or even obliteration of the marrow cavity. The affected bones are brittle and fractures occur with relatively slight stress. Marrow spaces not obliterated by bone overgrowth are frequently fibrotic and devoid of hematopoietic elements; thus, anemia associated with extramedullary hematopoiesis (hepatosplenomegaly) results. (REF. 1, p. 1321)

539. E. Aseptic necrosis may affect the tibial tubercle (Osgood-Schlatter's disease); navicular bone (Köhler's disease); and head of femur (Legg-Calvé-Perthes disease). (REF. 2, p. 1763)

540. C. In Ollier's disease the enchondromas (benign cartilaginous tumors within medullary cavity of bone) are randomly scattered throughout the skeletal system. The most common sites are the ends of long bones. Despite the morphologic similarity to Maffucci's syndrome, there is no evidence that Ollier's disease is genetic or hereditary. (REF. 2, pp. 1792–1793)

541. A. Osteomalacia is the most common remediable systemic bone disorder of the elderly. It is characterized by inadequate mineralization of bone matrix with resultant relative increase in the amount of osteoid and a decrease in appositional growth rate. The following are some of the causes of osteomalacia: (1) vitamin D deficiency; (2) impaired metabolism of vitamin D; (3) end-organ unresponsiveness; (4) renal phosphate leak; and (5) hereditary deficiency of alkaline phosphatase. (REF. 1, pp. 409–411)

542. D. Paget's disease is characterized by an initial excessive, haphazard, osteoclastic bone resorption followed by an osteoblastic response with the deposition of irregular woven bone. The bone replacement is not complete, some of the resorbed bone being replaced by highly vascularized connective tissue. The tilelike or mosaic pattern which is pathognomonic of Paget's disease results from the delayed mineralization of the newly laid down matrix causing persistence of the osteoid seams at the margins of the new bone. (REF. 1, pp. 1331–1332)

543. B. Colloid cysts (paraphyseal cysts) are limited to the roof of the third ventricle, midway between the interventricular foramina. At autopsy the incidence (2% of all intracranial tumors) exceeds the clinical incidence (0.5%) because only a fourth of these neoplasms reach the clinically significant size of 1 cm. Two types of ependyma-lined cysts, containing gelatinous grayish material, are identified. The more frequent type arises after the closure of the ependymal pouch; here, the cuboidal to columnar cells are ciliated. The other type is believed to be the result of the persistence of embryonic paraphyseal pouch; the cells are not ciliated. (REF. 2, p. 1923)

544. B. See explanatory answer 543. (REF. 2, p. 1923)

545. A. Neurilemmomas (Schwannomas) are neoplasms arising from Schwann cells and comprise 8% of all intracranial neoplasms. the most common site is the vestibular portion of the eighth nerve in the region of the internal acoustic meatus, growing into the cerebellopontine angle. The other nerves of origin in decreasing order of frequency are the ninth, seventh, eleventh, fifth, and fourth. (REF. 2, p. 1925)

546. A. See explanatory answer 545. (REF. 2, p. 1925)

547. C. Craniopharyngiomas (Rathke's pouch tumor, supracellular cyst) comprise 3% of all intracranial neoplasms. They seem to arise from squamous cell remnants of Rathke's pouch (Erdheim cell rests) that can be found at any level from the nasopharynx to the arachnoid covering the mammillary bodies. The peaks of incidence are in late childhood and early adulthood, and in the fifth decade. (REF. 2, p. 1922)

548. D. Sturge-Weber-Dimitri disease is a rare developmental anomaly of blood vessels in the brain and skin. There is a striking increase in blood vessels, many of which are collagenized, in the leptomeninges and atrophic portions of the brain (mainly the parietal and occipital lobes). Mineralization of cortical vessels gives the characteristic x-ray picture. The associated skin lesion consists of a "port-wine stain" nevus in the distribution of one or more branches of the trigeminal nerve. (REF. 2, pp. 1927–1928)

549. E. Déjerine-Sottas disease is a rare disorder producing enlargement of motor and sensory nerves, characterized by "onion-bulb" neuropathy. This reactive change, however, is not a specific change; it can occur in any chronic peripheral neuropathy that has recurrent episodes of demyelination and remyelination. (REF. 2, pp. 1935–1936)

550. C. Cyanotic congenital heart disease is associated with a high incidence of cerebral abscesses and is thought to be due to a right-to-left shunt and loss of filtering ability of the lungs for organisms. Other causes are direct implantation of microorganisms by surgery or trauma, by extension from a focus of infection in neighboring structures (mastoiditis), and by hematogenous spread from other organs. (REF. 1, pp. 1381–1382)

551. A. Also referred to as subacute spongiform encephalopathy and transmissible viral dementia, Creutzfeldt-Jacob disease is caused by transmissible agents with a long (months to years) incubation period. The brain characteristically shows "holes and bubbles" (status spongiosus) in the cortex. The holes appear on electron microscopy as intracytoplasmic membrane-bound vacuoles in neuronal and glial processes. There is little, if any, gross atrophy of the brain. The patients typically present with changes in personality and disturbance of spatial/visual coordination soon followed by progressive dementia with myoclonus, and eventually, death. The average duration of the illness is 7 months. (REF. 1, p. 1385)

552. E. Ninety-five percent of ruptured aneurysms are of the developmental (berry, saccular, "congenital") type; in 20%–30% of cases, there is more than one aneurysm. Most berry aneurysms bleed into the subarachnoid space and, to a lesser extent, into the adjacent intracerebral tissue. (REF. 1, p. 1393)

553. B. Alzheimer's disease is a degenerative disorder of unknown etiology. It is characterized by progressive global cerebral atrophy more marked in the frontal, parietal, and occipital cortices. Generally becoming apparent between 50 and 60 years of age, the disease characteristically progresses steadily over a span of 5–10 years resulting in severe dementia and death. Recent evidence suggests abnormalities in the presynaptic cholinergic system in the cortex which appear to correlate with the morphologic abnormalities. However, the cause of the cholinergic system abnormality is still unknown. (REF. 1, p. 1414)

554. D. Hemorrhage into the brain substance is most commonly caused by hypertensive vascular disease. Although the mechanism of hypertensive cerebral hemorrhage is not understood, the following facts are generally accepted: (1) it occurs in patients who have had significant systolic and diastolic elevations for at least several years, (2) the occurrence of hemorrhage is usually related to at least mild exertion, and (3) hemorrhage almost never happens in sleep. (REF. 1, p. 1392)

555. D. It has been postulated that intracerebral hemorrhage is precipitated by arteriolar necrosis or rupture of microaneurysms of small arteries (Charcot-Bouchard aneurysms). Intracerebral hemorrhage almost never occurs during sleep; it is usually associated with some form of exertion. (REF. 1, p. 1392)

11 Case Studies

Case 1 (Questions 556–559): Microscopic section of the kidney of a 60-year-old woman with azotemia and retinopathy (Figure 11.1).

556. The most likely diagnosis is
  - A. renal amyloidosis
  - B. focal embolic glomerulonephritis
  - C. the kidney in systemic lupus erythematosus
  - D. diabetes mellitus
  - E. the kidney in polyarteritis nodosa

557. Other lesions found in the kidney in this disease are
  - A. "wire-loop" lesions
  - B. necrotizing arteritis
  - C. protein casts in renal tubules with giant-cell reaction
  - D. glycogen vacuoles in renal tubules
  - E. hyperplastic arteriosclerosis

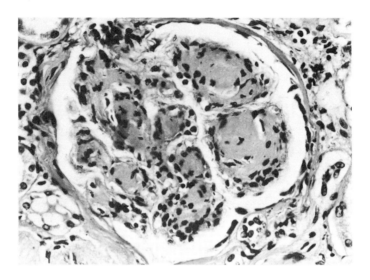

Figure 11.1

558. Laboratory diagnosis for this disease should include
  A. glucose tolerance test
  B. serum electrophoresis
  C. urine electrophoresis
  D. blood culture
  E. demonstration of antinuclear antibodies in the serum

559. All of the following are true of this lesion EXCEPT
  A. it is the most pathognomonic lesion in this disease
  B. it may manifest clinically as nephrotic syndrome
  C. it is often associated with necrotizing vasculitis
  D. this lesion is present in the mesangium of the renal glomeruli
  E. it is progressive in nature

Case 2 (Questions 560–565): A 59-year-old New York City resident presented with progressive dyspnea on exertion. He had smoked two packs of cigarettes a day for the past 20 years. On examination he had distended neck veins on expiration; the chest was barrel shaped, fixed in a hyperinflated inspiratory position, and was hyperresonant to percussion. There was restriction of diaphragmatic motion. The pulmonary second sound was prominent and split on expiration. Occasional expiratory wheezing was present. There was no history of chronic cough, expectoration of sputum, or recurrent fever.

560. The lung would most likely reveal
    A. chronic bronchitis
    B. bronchiectasis
    C. panacinar emphysema
    D. centriacinar emphysema
    E. bronchial asthma

561. Which of the following is LEAST likely to be present in this disease?
    A. Decreased vital capacity
    B. Decreased timed vital capacity
    C. Decreased maximal midexpiratory rate
    D. Decreased diffusing capacity
    E. Increased functional residual volume

562. This disease is NOT characterized by
    A. hypoxemia
    B. hypercapnia
    C. secondary polycythemia
    D. respiratory acidosis
    E. severe diffusion abnormalities

563. The earliest pathologic alteration in the pulmonary vasculature in this disease is
    A. intimal thickening of muscular arteries
    B. medial hypertrophy of muscular arteries
    C. arterialization of arterioles
    D. necrotizing vasculitis
    E. angiomatoid lesion of the muscular arteries

564. The most important pathogenetic lesion in this condition is
    A. chronic inflammation within the walls of bronchioles
    B. interstitial fibrosis
    C. acute bronchiolitis
    D. hyperplasia of bronchial mucous glands
    E. hypertrophy of bronchial smooth muscle

565. Predisposing and etiologic factors in this disease would include all of the following EXCEPT
- **A.** cigarette smoking
- **B.** atmospheric pollution
- **C.** alpha-1-antitrypsin deficiency
- **D.** chronic bronchitis
- **E.** acute staphylococcal pneumonia

Case 3 (Questions 566–569): A 32-year-old man, with known hypertension, presented with blurred vision. While in the emergency room he had multiple episodes of convulsion. His blood pressure was 220/150, his temperature and pulse were normal. Funduscopy revealed papilledema.

566. This illness may be caused by all of the following EXCEPT
- **A.** acute pyelonephritis
- **B.** chronic pyelonephritis
- **C.** acute glomerulonephritis
- **D.** chronic glomerulonephritis
- **E.** renovascular stenosis

567. Macroscopically, the kidney characteristically shows
- **A.** fine granularity
- **B.** coarse granularity
- **C.** "flea bites"
- **D.** multicystic change
- **E.** a waxy appearance

568. The most characteristic histopathological change in this disease is
- **A.** hyaline arteriosclerosis
- **B.** nodular glomerulosclerosis
- **C.** diffuse glomerulosclerosis
- **D.** hyperplastic arteriolosclerosis
- **E.** arterionephrosclerosis

569. If, at the time of death, this patient was NOT in congestive heart failure, the heart at autopsy would reveal

 A. left ventricular dilatation
 B. left ventricular hypertrophy
 C. right ventricular dilatation
 D. right ventricular hypertrophy
 E. combination of both dilatation and hypertrophy in the left ventricle

Case 4 (Questions 570–574): A 25-year-old nurse presented with malaise, lassitude, and easy fatigability that had lasted about 2 weeks. Two years previously she was hospitalized for jaundice, which resolved uneventfully on bed rest. Laboratory data revealed a total bilirubin of 3.0 g/100 ml, slightly elevated SGOT, SGPT, and alkaline phosphatase. Antismooth muscle antibody was elevated; antinuclear antibodies were present in the serum. Physical examination showed a mildly enlarged tender liver. Figure 11.2 shows the salient histopathologic changes.

Figure 11.2

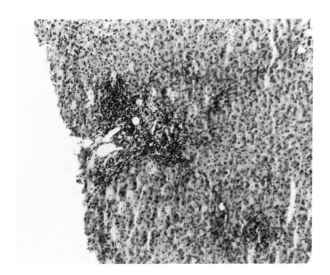

570. The most probable diagnosis is
    A. acute viral hepatitis
    B. chronic persistent hepatitis
    C. chronic active hepatitis
    D. cholestatic hepatitis
    E. submassive hepatic necrosis

571. This disease may progress to
    A. micronodular (regular) cirrhosis
    B. postnecrotic (irregular) cirrhosis
    C. biliary cirrhosis
    D. pigment cirrhosis
    E. none of the above

572. Which of the following tests would be most appropriate in this case?
    A. Alpha-fetoprotein
    B. Carcinoembryonic antigen
    C. Antimitochondrial antibody
    D. Hepatitis-associated antigen
    E. Antibody to hepatitis-associated antigen

573. Which of the following is most likely to produce a similar histologic appearance to the disease illustrated?
    A. Carbon tetrachloride poisoning
    B. Mushroom (*Amanita phalloides*) poisoning
    C. Alpha-methyldopa
    D. Contraceptive pills
    E. Yellow fever

574. "Piecemeal" necrosis of periportal hepatocytes is one of the characteristic features of
    A. chronic active hepatitis
    B. chronic persistent hepatitis
    C. sarcoidosis involving the liver
    D. acute leptospiral liver disease
    E. acute viral hepatitis

Case 5 (Questions 575–577): A 60-year-old woman was admitted because of spastic ataxic paraparesis. This complaint started 8 months previously as increased clumsiness on walking, followed by progressive weakness and paresthesias in the lower extremities. The myelogram showed a mass displacing the cord at level D8-9 vertebrae. This mass was subsequently removed and the histologic morphology is illustrated in Figure 11.3.

575. The histological type of this tumor is
   A. psammomatous
   B. meningotheliomatous
   C. fibroblastic
   D. ependymomatous
   E. none of the above

Figure 11.3

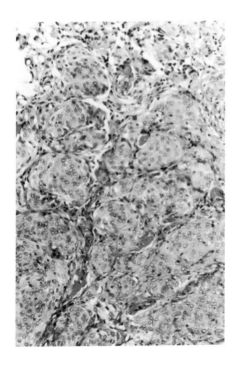

576. Hyperostosis associated with the tumor illustrated in Figure 11.3 is indicative of
   A. malignant degeneration of the tumor
   B. osseous invasion by a primary malignant tumor
   C. an independent tumor of the bone
   D. osseous metaplasia in the tumor
   E. none of the above

577. If this tumor (Figure 11.3) is located at the cerebellopontine angle, the most probable diagnosis is
   A. acoustic neuroma
   B. meningioma
   C. craniopharyngioma
   D. pinealoma
   E. ependymoma

Case 6 (Questions 578–582): A 32-year-old woman was admitted because of severe vaginal bleeding. She claimed to have been in good health until two months ago when she noticed progressive dysmenorrhea, menometrorrhagia, leukorrhea, and dyspareunia. The latter was accompanied by postcoital vaginal bleeding.

Examination: She was pale and diaphoretic. Her blood pressure was 80/40 mm/Hg; pulse, 140/min; and respiration 20/min. The other pertinent findings were a fairly nodular uterus, which was enlarged to 2–3 months gestation, and a large, mobile, bleeding ulcerated round tumor filling the proximal one-third of the vaginal canal. Flat films of the abdomen showed phylactenoid opacities.

Laboratory Data: Laboratory evaluation disclosed the following pertinent findings: hemoglobin 8 g/100 ml; hematocrit 23%; MCV 72 μ^3. Leukocytes 13,000/mm^3 with a normal differential. Pregnancy test was negative.

Hospital Course: Because of continued bleeding from the previously described mass, an abdominal hysterectomy was performed (Figure 11.4). The postoperative course was uneventful.

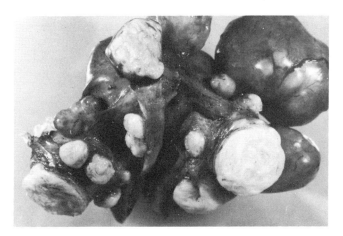

Figure 11.4

578. The most important microscopic criterion for the diagnosis of malignancy in this tumor is the
    A. presence of hermorrhage
    B. number of mitotic figures
    C. amount of bizarre cells
    D. degree of cellularity
    E. presence of focal degeneration

579. When these tumors are found in the stomach they are usually
    A. subserosal
    B. solitary
    C. large
    D. located at the antrum
    E. ulcerated

580. The hematologic picture was that of
    A. macrocytic normochromic anemia
    B. microcytic hypochromic anemia
    C. microcytic normochromic anemia
    D. macrocytic hypochromic anemia
    E. normocytic hypochromic anemia

581. If the patient had decreased serum iron and increased serum iron-binding capacity and had evidence of chronic infection without history of bleeding, a sensitive test would be bone marrow stained with
   A. Prussian blue
   B. H and E (hematoxylin and eosin)
   C. Congo red
   D. trichrome
   E. PAS (periodic acid-Schiff)

582. All of the following may produce uterine enlargement EXCEPT
   A. endometrial adenocarcinoma
   B. uterine adenomyosis
   C. uterine leiomyoma
   D. endometrial polyps
   E. myometrial hypertrophy

Case 7 (Questions 583–586): A 20-year-old female sought gynecologic consultation because of menometrorrhagia. A left ovarian mass (Figure 11.5) was discovered during pelvic examination.

583. This neoplasm is of
   A. undetermined origin
   B. Müllerian origin
   C. germ-cell origin
   D. germ-cell and stromal origin
   E. stromal origin

584. Figure 11.5 is a classic example of
   A. metastatic epidermoid carcinoma in an ovarian teratoma
   B. embryonal teratoma of ovary
   C. ovarian teratoma with a malignant component of epidermoid carcinoma
   D. cystic teratoma of ovary
   E. struma ovarii in an ovarian teratoma

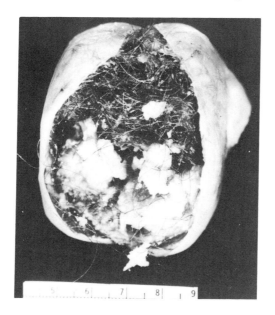

Figure 11.5

585. The tissue rarely encountered in this neoplasm is
    A. brain
    B. thyroid
    C. nerve
    D. liver
    E. skin appendage

586. All of the following statements concerning this tumor are true EXCEPT
    A. the sebaceous secretion is liquid at body temperature and tends to solidify on removal
    B. it is usually unilateral
    C. the most common malignant change is epidermoid carcinoma
    D. if it is ruptured, the greasy fluid provokes a predominant fibroblastic peritonitis resulting in nodules simulating metastatic cancer
    E. prognosis is poor if peritoneal implants are exclusively composed of mature glial tissue

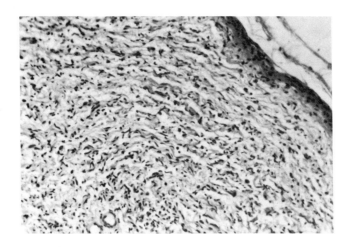

Figure 11.6

587. The lesion illustrated in Figure 11.6 is diagnostic of
  A. histiocytic lymphoma
  B. neurofibroma
  C. leiomyosarcoma
  D. malignant fibrous histiocytoma
  E. hemangiopericytoma

Questions 588 and 589 (Figure 11.7):

588. The histologic morphology in Figure 11.7 is diagnostic of
  A. anaplastic carcinoma
  B. lymphocytic lymphosarcoma, well differentiated
  C. Burkitt's tumor
  D. seminoma
  E. sarcoidosis

589. This lesion is characterized by all of the following EXCEPT
  A. it is related to Epstein-Barr virus
  B. it occurs predominantly as an extranodal disease
  C. it responds well to aggressive chemotherapy
  D. the lesion is derived from a clone of T lymphocytes
  E. the disease is endemic in Central Africa

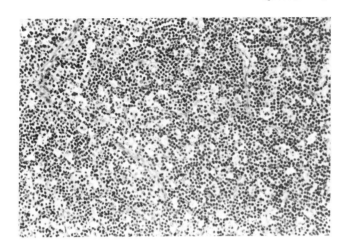

Figure 11.7

590. Figure 11.8 illustrates histological sections from the breast of a 52-year-old woman with an indurated mass. The most appropriate diagnosis is
   A. carcinoma
   B. adenosis
   C. fibrocystic disease
   D. papillomatosis
   E. none of the above

Figure 11.8

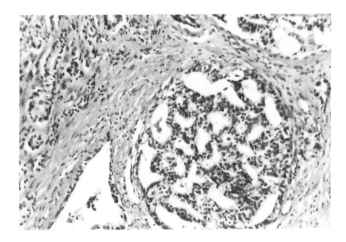

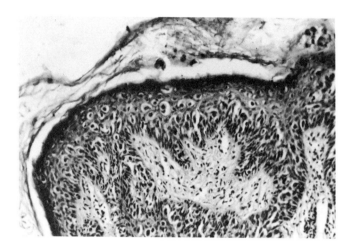

Figure 11.9

591. Figure 11.9 illustrates the histology of the biopsy of an excoriated, eczematoid lesion of the nipple of a 60-year-old woman. The photomicrograph is diagnostic of
    A. actinic keratosis
    B. pseudoepitheliomatous hyperplasia
    C. squamous carcinoma
    D. Paget's disease of the nipple
    E. lentigo maligna

592. This pericardial lesion (Figure 11.10) will most likely be encountered in
    A. tuberculosis
    B. congestive cardiomyopathy
    C. hypertensive heart disease
    D. acute rheumatic carditis
    E. syphilitic heart disease

593. Microscopic examination of this laryngeal lesion (Figure 11.11) is most likely to show
    A. squamous papillomatosis
    B. laryngeal polyp
    C. squamous cell carcinoma
    D. adenocarcinoma
    E. small cell anaplastic carcinoma

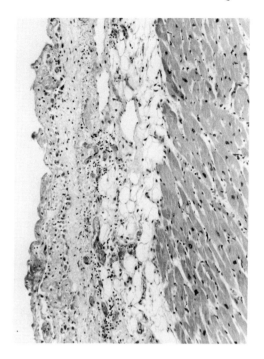

Figure 11.10

594. Photomicrographs from a "cold" thyroid nodule (Figure 11.12) in a 22-year-old woman. The most appropriate diagnosis is
    A. papillary carcinoma
    B. papillary adenoma
    C. papillary hyperplasia in a goiter
    D. papillo-follicular adenoma
    E. pseudo papillary formation in a thyroid adenoma

595. Figure 11.13 shows a hysterectomy specimen from a 25-year-old black woman with retained products of conception, rapidly enlarging uterus, and markedly elevated human chorionic gonadotropin titers. This tumor most likely originated from
    1. the ovary
    2. placental tissue
    3. the myocardium
    4. the endometrium
    5. fetal tissues

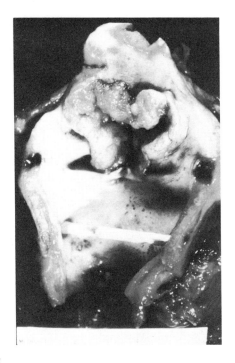

Figure 11.11

Figure 11.12

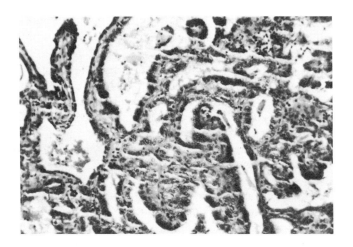

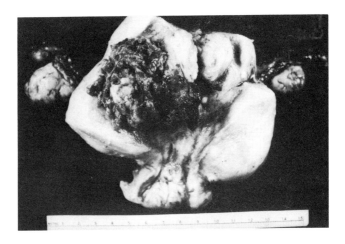

Figure 11.13

596. Which of the following statements concerning this tumor is incorrect?
    A. A tumor of similar histology and immunocytochemical characteristics may occur in men
    B. The tumor grows rapidly and frequently disseminates to distant organs
    C. Hydatidiform mole antedates this tumor in about half of patients
    D. Histological diagnosis rests on the demonstration of tissues derived from at least two germ layers
    E. Much more common in Oriental, Mexican, and African than in American women

597. Figure 11.14 shows the cut surface of the liver of a 35-year-old man. Etiologic considerations of the hepatic lesion should include all of the following EXCEPT
    A. chronic alcoholism
    B. protein-calorie malnutrition
    C. alpha-1-antitrypsin deficiency
    D. hepatolenticular degeneration (Wilson's disease)
    E. prolonged intake of alpha methyldopa

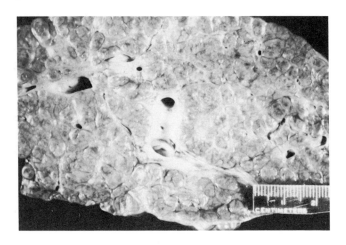

Figure 11.14

598. The spleen of this patient will manifest all of the following EXCEPT
   A. moderate to massive enlargement
   B. sinusoidal dilatation and congestion
   C. foci of fibrosis with iron deposits (Gandy-Gamna nodules)
   D. extramedullary hematopoeisis
   E. subcapsular infarcts

599. The lesion shown in the lateral wall of the left ventricle in Figure 11.15 is most consistent with
   A. myocarditis
   B. hemangioma
   C. acute myocardial infarct
   D. metastatic carcinoma
   E. none of the above

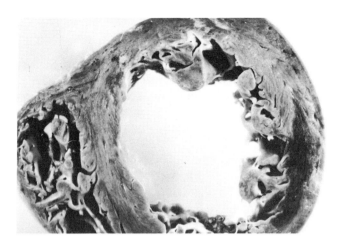

Figure 11.15

600. Microscopic section of the lesion illustrated in Figure 11.15 most likely will show which of the following?
   A. Malignant epithelial cells
   B. Necrosis of myocardial fibers and acute inflammation
   C. Fibrosis
   D. Diffused lymphocytic infiltrate with giant cells
   E. Predominantly proliferating capillaries

Answers and Comments

556. D. The lesion is nodular glomerulosclerosis, the most pathognomonic glomerular lesion in diabetes mellitus. The nodules are PAS-positive, contain mucopolysaccharides, and fibrils and have the same composition as the matrix deposits of diffuse glomerulosclerosis. (REF. 1, p. 1023)

557. D. These are otherwise called Armanni-Ebstein lesions. The only common condition in which it occurs is diabetes mellitus. It may be present in the glycogen storage diseases. (REF. 2, p. 1250)

558. A. A 2-hour postprandial blood glucose is also quite useful in confirming diabetes mellitus. (REF. 3, p. 172)

559. C. Kimmelstiel-Wilson syndrome comprises diabetes mellitus, hypertension, albuminuria, and edema. The most common histologic abnormality in this syndrome is diffuse glomerulosclerosis. Nodular glomerulosclerosis may be present. (REF. 1, p. 1023)

560. C. Some authorities believe that centriacinar emphysema is symptomless. In London, centriacinar emphysema is found in one of five fluid-fixed lungs of persons with normal chest x-rays without clinical lung disease. (REF. 1, pp. 717–718)

561. D. The diagnosis of chronic airway obstruction may be confirmed by utilizing the spirometric demonstrations of impaired air flow and increased airway resistance. (REF. 2, p. 906)

562. E. Emphysema is characterized by hypoventilation and CO_2 retention leading to respiratory acidosis, low pH, and elevated pCO_2. (REF. 2, p. 906)

563. B. These are all lesions of mild-to-moderate pulmonary hypertension. Severe lesions include angiomatoid and glomoid lesions and necrotizing vasculitis. (REF. 2, p. 866)

564. A. The essential lesion underlying emphysema is chronic inflammation within the walls of and around the terminal bronchioles. These become thickened, rigid, and narrowed, causing trapping of air in expiration and distention of the alveoli. (REF. 2, p. 903)

565. E. Pulmonary emphysema associated with alpha-1-antitrypsin deficiency occurs in patients homozygous for the deficiency. Its onset is in early adult life. The lower lobes are more severely affected than the upper lobes. The enzyme deficiency may also be associated with liver cirrhosis. (REF. 2, p. 904)

566. A. The symptoms and signs of this disease are those of malignant hypertension. Acute pyelonephritis is not known to cause hypertension. Approximately 90%–95% of hypertension is of uncertain origin (primary or essential). The remainder, called secondary, may be caused by the following, among others: polycystic kidneys, coarctation of the aorta, pheochromocytoma, hyperaldosteronism, and Cushing's syndrome. (REF. 2, pp. 752–754)

567. C. "Flea bites" refer to small pinpoint petechial hemorrhages that appear on the renal cortical surface. Although characteristic of malignant hypertension, a similar gross appearance may be seen in polyarteritis nodosa. (REF. 2, p. 754)

568. D. In addition to hyperplastic arteriolosclerosis, there may be necrotizing arteriolitis. An immunologic etiology is suggested for the latter. (REF. 2, p. 752)

569. B. Hypertension leads to concentric cardiac hypertrophy. In the decompensated patient with symptoms and signs of left heart failure, the left ventricle undergoes dilation. (REF. 2, p. 751)

570. C. The morphologic features are those of chronic active (aggressive) hepatitis. The portal tracts are enlarged and exhibit piecemeal necrosis. In addition, focal lobular necrosis may be present. Many patients, in time, would develop postnecrotic cirrhosis. The etiology and pathogenesis of chronic active hepatitis are poorly understood. While in some it may represent persistence or recurrence of viral infection, in others it may be an immune reaction of the cell-mediated or humoral type. This disease should be distinguished from chronic persistent hepatitis, which offers a better prognosis. (REF. 1, pp. 907–909)

571. B. Postnecrotic cirrhosis, sometimes called irregular cirrhosis, is characterized by distortion of normal lobular hepatic architecture; nodules of regeneration, ranging up to 5 cm in diameter, are separated by thick fibrous bands, which may contain variable amounts of chronic inflammatory cells. Other morphologic features that may be present include bile duct proliferation, cholestasis and focal necrosis. The etiology of postnecrotic cirrhosis may be viral (type B or type non-A, non-B), autoimmune (lupoid), or toxin and drug-induced. (REF. 1, pp. 923–924)

572. D. Hepatitis-associated antigen may also be demonstrated in the perinuclear cytoplasm of hepatocytes using various stains, one of which is the immunoperoxidase technique. (REF. 1, p. 902)

573. C. Carbon tetrachloride usually causes centrolobular necrosis, contraceptive pills simple cholestasis, and yellow fever predominantly midzonal necrosis. Alpha methyldopa, however, may cause a disease indistinguishable from viral hepatitis, which may proceed to chronic active hepatitis. (REF. 1, pp. 450–451)

574. A. In addition, chronic active hepatitis, shows enlargement of portal tracts by chronic inflammatory cells, focal lobular necrosis, and elevated gamma globulin. Four variants of this entity are recognized based on subtle differences in clinical patterns. (REF. 1, p. 907)

575. B. The endotheliomatous, or meningotheliomatous, meningioma consists of clusters of cells with varying amounts of stroma. These cells are polygonal and epithelial-like with ill-defined cell borders and pale cytoplasm. They have moderately chromatic oval or round nuclei. The stroma is collagenous or hyalinized and contains large numbers of blood vessels. The predominant pattern is a whorling effect where the cells are closely wrapped around one another. (REF. 1, p. 1409)

576. E. Malignant transformation of a meningioma has been described and may occur as an exceptional event. A truly malignant lesion produces osteoclastic rather than osteoblastic change.

Invasion of bone is not of itself indicative of malignancy; for example, meningiomas en plaque spread along the deeper surface of the dura and tend to invade the overlying bone, producing hyperostosis. (REF. 1, p. 1409)

577. B. The histologic picture illustrated in Figure 11.3 is that of a meningotheliomatous meningioma. Although a less common location, the posterior fossa (cerebellopontine angle) is one of the anatomic sites of meningioma. The location of acoustic neuroma in the angle formed by the pons, medulla, and cerebellum accounts for the commonly used synonym of "cerebellopontine angle" tumors. (REF. 2, p. 1924)

578. B. Tumors with fewer than five mitoses per high-power field, in the most active areas, behave practically always as benign tumors even in the presence of atypical cells, hyperchromatic nuclei, and multinucleated forms. Tumors with 10 or more mitoses per high-power field behave as malignant neoplasms regardless of how innocuous the microscopic appearance is. (REF. 1, p. 1140)

579. E. Leiomyomas are the most common benign tumors of the stomach. They are often multiple, form small well-defined homogeneous nodules, appear most commonly in the fundus, are submucosal (about 60%), and grow into the lumen of the stomach. (REF. 1, p. 820)

580. B. The MCV of 72 μ^3 and the MCHC of 25% point to hypochromic microcytic anemia that resulted from the continued loss of blood. (REF. 3, pp. 696–697)

581. A. Lack of hemosiderin in the marrow is a sensitive indicator of iron deficiency. Prussian blue stains the iron marrow content. (REF. 1, p. 656)

582. D. Although endometrial polyps are multicentric in origin, they are usually small sessile projecting masses, and do not produce uterine enlargement. (REF. 1, p. 1135)

583. C. Like dysgerminoma, endodermal sinus tumor, primary choriocarcinoma of ovary, embryonal carcinoma, and adult solid teratoma, cystic teratoma, is of germ-cell origin. (REF. 1, p. 1149)

584. D. Characteristically, cystic teratomas are unilocular thin-walled cysts within a smooth glistening serosa. An admixture of matted strands of hair and thick yellow-white sebaceous material fill the lumen. Adult teratomas contain thyroid tissue in approximately 12%-15% of cases; however, the diagnosis of struma ovarii should not be made unless the thyroid tissue predominates or if there is evidence of either neoplasia or hormonal function. Classically, teratomas are brown in color and spongy in consistency. (REF. 1, pp. 1149–1150)

585. D. Kidney and liver tissue occur rarely, if at all. Skin appendages are extremely common; brain and nerve tissue occur frequently; and thyroid tissue is found in about 12%–15% of cases. (REF. 1, pp. 1149–1150)

586. E. Adult teratomas of both the cystic and solid variety, especially the latter, are occasionally accompanied by peritoneal implants. If these are purely mature glial tissue the prognosis is excellent. Conversely, if other tissues such as epithelium are present, the prognosis is poor. (REF. 1, pp. 1149–1151)

587. B. The photomicrograph shows the characteristic features of a neurofibroma. In von Recklinghausen's disease, multiple neurofibromas of the skin, sympathetic chain and motor and sensory nerve trunks are associated with café-au-lait spots. The typical skin lesion is circumscribed. The tumor cells are fusiform and usually twisted, and are separated by an intercellular matrix composed of fibrocollagenous tissue. (REF. 1, p. 1432)

588. C. Burkitt's tumor, first described as an extranodal (facial) malignant lymphoma in African children, occurs most frequently between the ages of 3 and 12 years. In American patients, abdominal and pelvic involvement is predominant. Histologically, the tumor is composed of undifferentiated lymphoid cells with pyroninophilic cytoplasm. Scattered among the tumor cells are pale vacuolated histiocytes, giving rise to the characteristic "starry-sky" appearance. (REF. 1, pp. 662–663)

589. D. Epstein-Barr virus has also been implicated, less convincingly, however, in undifferentiated nasopharyngeal carcinoma. (REF. 1, p. 245)

590. A. The main lesion consists of an intraductal carcinoma which shows characteristic cribriform pattern composed of small, round cells. Surrounding this is an infiltrating adenocarcinoma of the breast. (REF. 1, p. 1181)

591. D. The characteristic histologic appearance of Paget's disease of the nipple, showing the invasion of the epidermis by innumerable large cells with clear cytoplasm and abnormal hyperchromatic nuclei, is illustrated. The large, anaplastic, vacuolated cells in the epidermis are mucicarminophilic. This lesion is now accepted as an invasion of the epidermis by the tumor cells from an underlying intraductal carcinoma. By contrast, Paget's disease of the vulva is not associated with an underlying adenocarcinoma in up to one-third of the cases. (REF. 1, p. 1181)

592. D. The histological changes are those of fibrinous pericarditis. Scattered lymphocytes and reactive mesothelial cells are entrapped in the lesion. Tuberculosis typically manifests granulomatous pericarditis. The pericardium is usually unaffected in congestive cardiomyopathy, hypertensive, or syphilitic heart disease. Because of its shaggy appearance, the fibrinous pericarditis of acute rheumatic carditis has been called "bread-and-butter" type pericarditis. (REF. 1, p. 573)

593. C. The gross photograph shows the characteristic appearance of carcinoma of the larynx. Squamous cell carcinoma of the larynx is the most common malignant epithelial neoplasm of the upper respiratory tract and is closely related to a history of chronic alcoholism and cigarette smoking. (REF. 5, pp. 509–511)

594. A. The papillary fronds, which are simple or complicated, are lined by single or multilayered atypical epithelial cells characteristic of a well-differentiated papillary carcinoma of the thyroid. The nuclei of the tumor cells show the so-called ground glass appearance. (REF. 1, pp. 1219–1220)

595. B. The clincal history and the gross pathologic features are typical of choriocarcinoma. The tumor is usually soft, bulky, and reveals extensive necrosis and hemorrhage. The effect of treatment and the extent of the disease can be monitored with the measurement of HCG titers. (REF. 1, pp. 1160–1162)

596. D. Identification of both cytotrophoblastic and syncytiotrophoblastic cells is important in the microscopic diagnosis of choriocarcinoma. The tumor cells are most frequently anaplastic but may be as differentiated as in the hydatidiform mole. The absence of chorionic villi distinguishes the choriocarcinoma. (REF. 1, pp. 1160, 1388)

597. B. The section shows typical features of mixed micronodular and macronodular cirrhosis, predominantly the latter. The liver of patients with protein-calorie malnutrition is usually fatty, a change presumed to result from decreased synthesis of protein carriers necessary for lipoprotein formation. These livers do not become cirrhotic. (REF. 1, pp. 402, 915–933)

598. E. Cirrhosis is the most common cause of striking congestive splenomegaly. Spleen weights of 100 g or more are not unusual. The spleen is firm in consistency and the cut surface appears meaty. Infarcts are not a feature of this type of splenic enlargement. (REF. 1, pp. 700–701)

599. C. The acute myocardial infarct shown in the photograph is about 2 to 3 days old. (REF. 1, p. 559)

600. B. A 2- to 3-day-old myocardial infarct is characterized by myocardial necrosis, fatty change, polymorphonuclear leukocytic infiltrate, and acute congestion at the periphery of the lesion. (REF. 1, pp. 559–561)

References

1. Robbins, S.L., Cotran, R.S., Kumar, V.: *Pathologic Basis of Disease*, 3rd Ed. W.B. Saunders, Philadelphia, 1984.

2. Kissane, J.M. (Ed): *Anderson's Pathology*, 8th Ed. C.V. Mosby, St. Louis, 1985.

3. Henry, J.B.: *Todd-Sanford-Davidsohn Clinical Diagnosis and Management by Laboratory Methods*, 17th Ed. W.B. Saunders, Philadelphia, 1984.

4. Jawetz, E., Melnick, J.L., Adelberg, E.A.: *Review of Medical Microbiology*, 17th Ed. Lange Medical Publications, Los Altos, Calif., 1987.

5. Silverberg, S.G. (Ed): *Principles and Practice of Surgical Pathology*. John Wiley and Sons, New York, 1983.

6. Robbins, S.L., Kumar, V.: *Basic Pathology*, 4th Ed. W.B. Saunders, Philadelphia, 1987.